Sarah B. Laditka, PhD
Editor

Health Expectations
for Older Women:
International Perspectives

Health Expectations for Older Women: International Perspectives
has been co-published simultaneously as *Journal of Women &
Aging*, Volume 14, Numbers 1/2 2002.

Pre-publication
REVIEWS,
COMMENTARIES,
EVALUATIONS . . .

"**B**RINGS TOGETHER NOTED
EXPERTS FROM AROUND
THE WORLD who shed new light on
how women age. . . . This volume is
sweeping in its coverage, including
specific analyses of the U.S., the U.K.,
Japan, Canada, The Netherlands, and
Fiji, as well as an overview of all 191
WHO member countries. A nice balance of country-specific and global
studies. . . . Gerontologists, epidemiologists, and demographers will find
the information presented to be TIMELY,
RIGOROUS, AND ACCESSIBLE."

Christine L. Himes, PhD,
Associate Professor of Sociology,
Syracuse University

"Women live longer than men but spend a greater proportion of their lives in poor health. This book BRINGS TOGETHER A NUMBER OF CUTTING-EDGE APPROACHES to the study of this, and related problems and paradoxes. The authors include many of the foremost researchers in the field. . . . OF GREAT VALUE to those interested in gender and health, those interested in trends and determinants of good health and mortality, and methodologists. Policymakers should also find this book of value, given the very important implications of variations in health expectations."

Emily Grundy, PhD
Reader in Social Gerontology and Head, Centre for Population Studies, London School of Hygiene and Tropical Medicine

"Excellent. . . . A MUST for scholars, health policy professionals, and individuals concerned with the lives of older women. The breadth of countries and international data sets and the array of health topics provide a foundation for understanding similarities and dissimilarities between older women. The sophisticated use of data and modeling techniques provides insight into the unique experiences of women in developed and developing countries."

Janice I. Farkas, PhD
Director, Gerontology Program University of North Carolina, Greensboro

"A WELCOME ADDITION to the interdisciplinary research literature on health and aging. . . . A well-written exploration of this critical topic. Policymakers, practitioners, planners, and family members throughout the world are grappling with the demographic *tsunami* of elderly women that will be hitting in the next two decades. With the help of this book, they can prepare to ride the wave."

Sharon Buchbinder, RN, PhD
Associate Professor and Coordinator, Health Care Management Program; Senior Editor, Research in Healthcare Financial Management, *Department of Health Science, Towson University*

Health Expectations
for Older Women:
International Perspectives

Health Expectations for Older Women: International Perspectives has been co-published simultaneously as *Journal of Women & Aging*, Volume 14, Numbers 1/2 2002.

The *Journal of Women & Aging* Monographic "Separates"

Below is a list of "separates," which in serials librarianship means a special issue simultaneously published as a special journal issue or double-issue *and* as a "separate" hardbound monograph. (This is a format which we also call a "DocuSerial.")

"Separates" are published because specialized libraries or professionals may wish to purchase a specific thematic issue by itself in a format which can be separately cataloged and shelved, as opposed to purchasing the journal on an on-going basis. Faculty members may also more easily consider a "separate" for classroom adoption.

"Separates" are carefully classified separately with the major book jobbers so that the journal tie-in can be noted on new book order slips to avoid duplicate purchasing.

You may wish to visit Haworth's website at . . .

http://www.HaworthPress.com

. . . to search our online catalog for complete tables of contents of these separates and related publications.

You may also call 1-800-HAWORTH (outside US/Canada: 607-722-5857), or Fax 1-800-895-0582 (outside US/Canada: 607-771-0012), or e-mail at:

getinfo@haworthpressinc.com

Health Expectations for Older Women: International Perspectives, edited by Sarah B. Laditka, PhD (Vol. 14, No. 1/2, 2002). *"BRINGS TOGETHER NOTED EXPERTS FROM AROUND THE WORLD who shed new light on how women age. . . . This volume is sweeping in its coverage, including specific analyses of the U.S., the U.K., Japan, Canada, The Netherlands, and Fiji, as well as an overview of all 191 WHO member countries. A nice balance of country-specific and global studies. . . . Gerontologists, epidemiologists, and demographers will find the information presented to be TIMELY, RIGOROUS, AND ACCESSIBLE." (Christine L. Himes, PhD, Associate Professor of Sociology, Syracuse University)*

Fundamentals of Feminist Gerontology, edited by J. Dianne Garner, DSW (Vol. 11, No. 2/3, 1999). *Strives to increase women's self-esteem and their overall quality of life by encouraging education and putting a stop to age, sex, and race discrimination.*

Old, Female, and Rural, edited by B. Jan McCulloch (Vol. 10, No. 4, 1998). *"An excellent job of bringing together experts from four different disciplines to illuminate the basic interdisciplinary nature of gerontology." (Dr. Jean Turner, Associate Professor, Human Development and Family Services, University of Arkansas, Fayetteville, Arkansas)*

Relationships Between Women in Later Life, edited by Karen A. Roberto (Vol. 8, No. 3/4, 1996). *"Provides an impressive array of issues about women's social networks. . . . Important, up-to-date empirical studies that will fill a significant gap in our understanding about the great diversity in the lives of older women today." (European Federation of the Elderly)*

Older Women with Chronic Pain, edited by Karen A. Roberto (Vol. 6, No. 4, 1994). *"Readers interested in the health concerns of older women, and older women themselves, will appreciate the insight and information in this book." (Feminist Bookstore News)*

Women and Healthy Aging: Living Productively in Spite of It All, edited by J. Dianne Garner and Alice A. Young (Vol. 5, No. 3/4, 1994). *"For those who are not aged themselves, it helps to bring about insights that are not possible when one holds the commonly taught view that disability of any degree is strictly debilitating." (Linda Vinton, PhD, Associate Professor, School of Social Work, Florida State University; Research Affiliate, Pepper Institute on Aging and Public Policy)*

Women in Mid-Life: Planning for Tomorrow, edited by Christopher L. Hayes (Vol. 4, No. 4, 1993). *"Contains illuminating insights into aspects of women's mid-life experiences." (Age and Ageing)*

Women, Aging and Ageism, edited by Evelyn Rosenthal (Vol. 2, No. 2, 1990). *"Readers should find this book helpful in gaining new insights to issues women face in old age . . . Enlightening."* *(Educational Gerontology)*

Women as They Age: Challenge, Opportunity, and Triumph, edited by J. Dianne Garner and Susan O. Mercer (Vol. 1, No. 1/2/3, 1989). *"Offers provocative insights into the strengths, dilemmas, and challenges confronting the current and future cohorts of older women."* *(Affilia: Journal of Women and Social Work)*

Indexing, Abstracting & Website/Internet Coverage

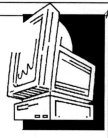

This section provides you with a list of major indexing & abstracting services. That is to say, each service began covering this periodical during the year noted in the right column. Most Websites which are listed below have indicated that they will either post, disseminate, compile, archive, cite or alert their own Website users with research-based content from this work. (This list is as current as the copyright date of this publication.)

Abstracting, Website/Indexing Coverage . . . . Year When Coverage Began

- *Abstracts in Anthropology* 1992
- *Abstracts in Social Gerontology: Current Literature on Aging* 1988
- *Academic ASAP <www.galegroup.com>* 1992
- *Academic Index (on-line)* 1992
- *Academic Search Elite (EBSCO)* 1996
- *AgeInfo CD-ROM* 1995
- *AgeLine Database* 1993
- *Behavioral Medicine Abstracts* 1992
- *Cambridge Scientific Abstracts (Health & Safety Science Abstracts)*
   <www.csa.com> 1993
- *CINAHL (Cumulative Index to Nursing & Allied Health*
   Literature), in print, EBSCO, and SilverPlatter, Data-Star,
   and PaperChase. (Support materials include Subject Heading
   List, Database Search Guide, and instructional video)
   <www.cinahl.com> 1997
- *CNPIEC Reference Guide: Chinese National Directory of Foreign*
   Periodicals 1995
- *Combined Health Information Database (CHID)* 1995

(continued)

(continued)

- *Periodical Abstracts Select (abstracting & indexing service covering most frequently requested journals in general reference, plus journals requested in libraries serving undergraduate programs, available from University Microfilms International (UMI), 300 North Zeeb Road, P.O. Box 1346, Ann Arbor, MI 48106-1346)* **1994**
- *Psychological Abstracts (PsycINFO) <www.apa.org>* **2002**
- *RESEARCH ALERT/ISI Alerting Services <www.isinet.com>* **1995**
- *Social Sciences Citation Index <www.isinet.com>* **1995**
- *Social Scisearch <www.isinet.com>* **1995**
- *Social Services Abstracts <www.csa.com>* **1992**
- *Social Work Abstracts <www.silverplatter.com/catalog/swab.htm>* . . . **1992**
- *Sociological Abstracts (SA) <www.csa.com>* **1992**
- *Studies on Women Abstracts <www.tandf.co.uk>* **1988**
- *SwetsNet <www.swetsnet.com>* **2002**
- *Women Studies Abstracts* **1991**
- *Women's Healthbeat* **1999**
- *Women's Studies Index (indexed comprehensively)* **1992**

Special Bibliographic Notes related to special journal issues (separates) and indexing/abstracting:

- indexing/abstracting services in this list will also cover material in any "separate" that is co-published simultaneously with Haworth's special thematic journal issue or DocuSerial. Indexing/abstracting usually covers material at the article/chapter level.
- monographic co-editions are intended for either non-subscribers or libraries which intend to purchase a second copy for their circulating collections.
- monographic co-editions are reported to all jobbers/wholesalers/approval plans. The source journal is listed as the "series" to assist the prevention of duplicate purchasing in the same manner utilized for books-in-series.
- to facilitate user/access services all indexing/abstracting services are encouraged to utilize the co-indexing entry note indicated at the bottom of the first page of each article/chapter/contribution.
- this is intended to assist a library user of any reference tool (whether print, electronic, online, or CD-ROM) to locate the monographic version if the library has purchased this version but not a subscription to the source journal.
- individual articles/chapters in any Haworth publication are also available through the Haworth Document Delivery Service (HDDS).

Health Expectations for Older Women: International Perspectives

Sarah B. Laditka, PhD
Editor

Health Expectations for Older Women: International Perspectives has been co-published simultaneously as *Journal of Women & Aging*, Volume 14, Numbers 1/2 2002.

The Haworth Press, Inc.
New York • London • Oxford

Health Expectations for Older Women: International Perspectives has been co-published simultaneously as *Journal of Women & Aging*™, Volume 14, Numbers 1/2 2002.

The development, preparation, and publication of this work has been undertaken with great care. However, the publisher, employees, editors, and agents of The Haworth Press and all imprints of The Haworth Press, Inc., including The Haworth Medical Press® and Pharmaceutical Products Press®, are not responsible for any errors contained herein or for consequences that may ensue from use of materials or information contained in this work. Opinions expressed by the author(s) are not necessarily those of The Haworth Press, Inc. With regard to case studies, identities and circumstances of individuals discussed herein have been changed to protect confidentiality. Any resemblance to actual persons, living or dead, is entirely coincidental.

The Haworth Press, Inc., 10 Alice Street, Binghamton, NY 13904-1580 USA

Cover design by Jennifer M. Gaska

Library of Congress Cataloging-in-Publication Data

Health expectations for older women : international perspectives / Sarah B. Laditka, editor.
     p. cm.
     "Co-published simultaneously as Journal of women & aging, vol. 14, nos. 1/2 2002"–T.p. verso.
     Includes bibliographical references and index.
     ISBN 0-7890-1926-4 (hard : alk. paper) – ISBN 0-7890-1927-2 (pbk. : alk. paper)
     1. Aged women–Health and hygiene–Longitudinal studies.
     [DNLM: 1. Women's Health– Aged. 2. Cross-Cultural Comparison–Aged. 3. Disabled Persons–Aged. 4. Life Expectancy.
     WA 309 H43425 2002] I. Laditka, Sarah B. II. Journal of women & aging.
RA564.85 .H399 2002
613'.0438–dc21
                                 2002008192

Health Expectations for Older Women: International Perspectives

CONTENTS

ABOUT THE EDITOR

Sarah B. Laditka, PhD, is Associate Professor of Health Services Management and Director of the Center for Health and Aging at the State University of New York Institute of Technology. Her previous positions include Manager of Health Programs at the General Electric Company, Health Care Coordinator for the Central New York Health Systems Agency, and Registered Nurse. Dr. Laditka's curent research focuses on healthy life expectancy, utilization, access, and quality of health services for special populations, and utilization of and satisfaction with long-term care services. She has presented numerous papers at regional, national, and international conferences. Dr. Laditka's research has been published in *Administration and Policy in Mental Health, Archives of Internal Medicine, Home Health Care Services Quarterly, Journal of Aging and Health, Journal of Applied Gerontology, Journal of Gerontology: Social Sciences, Journal of Health & Social Policy, Journal of Women & Aging, Policy Studies Review,* and *Research on Aging.*

Preface

This volume explores international trends in health and longevity with a special focus on older women. I hope readers will gain a richer understanding of women's health and the complex issues of life quality at older ages in many countries. In editing this volume, I have been privileged to work with a talented and diverse group of researchers from around the world and from a broad range of disciplines. Contributors include demographers, economists, epidemiologists, gerontologists, medical statisticians, policy analysts, physicians, public health directors, and sociologists. At the end of the volume, I have included a section *About the Contributors,* with information about each author. These researchers are related in their interest and enthusiasm to better understand the nature of longevity and health for older individuals. Demographic trends play a large role in shaping our world. They influence governments, non-government organizations, families, and the plans we all make for our own older age. These studies should be useful for practitioners, policymakers, researchers, and students interested in health and aging.

Sarah B. Laditka
Hamilton, NY
September 2001

[Haworth co-indexing entry note]: "Preface." Laditka, Sarah B. Co-published simultaneously in *Journal of Women & Aging* (The Haworth Press, Inc.) Vol. 14, No. 1/2, 2002, p. xvii; and: *Health Expectations for Older Women: International Perspectives* (ed: Sarah B. Laditka) The Haworth Press, Inc., 2002, p. xiii. Single or multiple copies of this article are available for a fee from The Haworth Document Delivery Service [1-800-HAWORTH 9:00 a.m. - 5:00 p.m. (EST). E-mail address: getinfo@haworthpressinc.com].

xiii

Introduction:
Health Expectations
for Older Women:
International Perspectives

Sarah B. Laditka, PhD

Dramatic life expectancy gains are among the greatest achievements of the twentieth century. For women, longer lives have brought important changes in work and retirement patterns, family life, and caregiving. Early in the century, most of the gains came from controlling infectious diseases and improving public health (Fuchs, 1974; Olshansky, Carnes, Rogers, & Smith, 1997). These gains brought additional years of good health. Beginning about three decades ago, death rates for fatal diseases often associated with older age fell considerably. This decline was particularly notable for cardiovascular diseases, such as stroke and heart disease (Davis et al., 1985; McGovern, Burke, Spafka, Folsom, & Blackburn, 1992). Reduced mortality from major fatal diseases brought even more years of life for the average individual. However, many researchers found that these longevity gains also brought additional years spent in worse health (Colvez & Blanchet, 1981; Crimmins, Saito, & Ingegneri, 1989). Thus, the demography of longevity and health has important implications for women of all ages: those who are

Sarah B. Laditka is Associate Professor of Health Services Management and Director of the Center for Health and Aging at the State University of New York Institute of Technology, P.O. Box 3050, Utica, NY 13504 (E-mail: laditks@sunyit.edu).

[Haworth co-indexing entry note]: "Introduction: Health Expectations for Older Women: International Perspectives." Laditka, Sarah B. Co-published simultaneously in *Journal of Women & Aging* (The Haworth Press, Inc.) Vol. 14, No. 1/2, 2002, pp. 1-7; and: *Health Expectations for Older Women: International Perspectives* (ed: Sarah B. Laditka) The Haworth Press, Inc., 2002, pp. 1-7. Single or multiple copies of this article are available for a fee from The Haworth Document Delivery Service [1-800-HAWORTH 9:00 a.m. - 5:00 p.m. (EST). E-mail address: getinfo@haworthpressinc.com].

old, a group that can, on average, anticipate many more years of life than most women of previous generations; those who are approaching old age and must plan for many years of continued work or lengthy retirement; younger women who care for aging parents informally; and the large corps of women who serve older persons in the formal health care system.

Another momentous epidemiological shift appears to have been underway during the past two decades, again with important implications for the lives of women. In the United States and a number of other developed countries, there is growing evidence that the proportion of the older population with severe disability has declined (Doblhammer & Kytir, 2001; Freedman & Martin, 1998; Manton, Corder, & Stallard, 1993). This decline in the prevalence of disability has been attributed to many factors, including better knowledge of healthy lifestyle choices, advances in medical treatment and technology, and prescription drugs (Rowe & Kahn, 1998; Vita, Terry, Hubert, & Fries, 1998). These dramatic changes in longevity *and* health at older ages have redefined how we conceive of old age. In response to a recent national poll of older people conducted for the National Institute on Aging, for example, almost 50% of people between ages 65 and 69, and nearly a third of those in their seventies, said they consider themselves middle-aged (Clendinen, 2000).

Policymakers, practitioners, and researchers agree that the demand for health care resources and expenditures for health care and other services for older people depends on both the number of older people and their health status (Jacobzone, 2000; Lubitz, Beebe, & Baker, 1995). But the relationship between changing disability levels and use of formal and informal services is complex. Use and cost outcomes will depend on many factors. Will current trends reducing the prevalence of disability continue? Will high costs of health care at older ages be avoided–or merely postponed to later life? At what rate will health care costs rise (Freudenheim, 2001; Hogan, Lunney, Gabel, & Lynn, 2001)? Only time will provide certain answers for these questions. But the extraordinary increase in life expectancy, and growth in the number of older people throughout the world, has made disability a pivotal factor for understanding health care resource needs and social system planning.

Increasingly, policymakers are using disability indicators as a measure of population health. One useful indicator of population health is "health expectancy." This indicator was first proposed by the U.S. Department of Health, Education, and Welfare (1969) about three decades ago, and has been adopted for use by the World Health Organization. To estimate health expectancy, researchers partition total life expectancy into two component parts. One part is healthy life expectancy, also often referred to as active life expectancy or disability free life expectancy. This component is a measure of the years an individual can expect to live free of disability. The second part measures the years a person can expect to live with disability, also commonly referred to as inactive life expectancy or disabled life expectancy.

Researchers are actively studying both healthy and disabled life expectancy. For example, an international group of research scientists, known as the International Network on Health Expectancy or REVES (Réseau Espérance de Vie en Santé), has developed and compared various measures of health expectancy across countries and time spans to evaluate changes in health expectancies among populations. Olshansky and Wilkins (1998) review the development of the REVES network. A comprehensive review and synthesis of research conducted by REVES network scientists during the past decade is provided in *Determining Health Expectancies* (in press).

VOLUME OVERVIEW

Studies included in this volume examine recent trends in health expectancies with a special focus on older women. Women comprise the majority of most older populations, and both the number of older women and their percentage of populations throughout the world will grow rapidly in the coming decades (Kinsella, 2000). Thus, health expectancy trends for women are particularly important. Authors for this volume were selected to represent a variety of developed countries, as well several perspectives about developing countries. These studies provide information that can be used by practitioners, policymakers, and researchers alike to help plan for a wide range of long-term care services and policies. These include services and policies that would assist older women and men, as well as their caregivers.

In the first study, Douglas A. Wolf, James N. Laditka, and I examine life expectancy and active life expectancy among older women distinguished by race, education, and marital status, from two perspectives. We examine the variability inherent in estimates of active and inactive life, and differences in active life expectancy among population subgroups. The results highlight the uncertainty associated with forecasting demand for long-term care services. The results also underscore the heterogeneity of disability in older populations, reinforcing the usefulness of separately estimating health expectancies among well-defined groups of older women.

This volume also includes two perspectives about gender differences in life expectancy associated with specific diseases. These perspectives are useful when evaluating research and policy options addressing various diseases, and also for projecting demand for health care services. Dorly J. H. Deeg, France Portrait, and Maarten Lindeboom use "health profiles," which group individuals based on the type and extent of health problems, to identify differences in disease types for older women and men in The Netherlands. Among the differences in the health profiles, older women are more likely to be cognitively disabled than older men, and also live longer with this disability. Using data from the United States, Eileen M. Crimmins, Jung Ki Kim, and Aaron Hagedorn examine health expectancy differences for six major diseases and two important health risk factors for older women and men. They find that women live longer than men with all major diseases studied, including heart disease, despite notably later disease onset. However, men are more likely to experience risk factors (being overweight and not seeing a physician on a regular basis) than women.

Gender differences for risk factors such as smoking and obesity and for several diseases are examined by Alain Bélanger, Laurent Martel, Jean-Marie Berthelot, and Russell Wilkins using data from Canada. They find individuals with diabetes or cancer live more disabled lives than those without these diseases. Using data from the United Kingdom, Carol Jagger and Fiona Matthews examine gender differences in functional, cognitive, and physical impairment, and the influence of missing data on impairment estimates. Their results show that women are substantially more likely than men to suffer from cognitive, physical, and functional impairments, particularly at older ages. Importantly, they find that excluding missing data, which is often present in large surveys of older people, is likely to result in underestimates of impairment for women and men.

Colin D. Mathers, Christopher J. L. Murray, Alan D. Lopez, Ritu Sadana, and Joshua A. Salomon present estimates of total, active, and disabled life expectancy for older women and men in many developing and developed countries. Dr. Mathers and his colleagues find women live notably longer in developed countries than in developing countries; for most countries studied, they also find there are substantial gender differences in healthy life expectancy and in the prevalence of specific diseases that cause disability. Jean-Marie Robine, Carol Jagger, and

Emmanuelle Cambois use data from the European Community Household Panel to examine gender differences in life expectancy and healthy life expectancy in twelve European countries. Although women live notably longer than men in all twelve countries, this research finds that the proportion of healthy life expectancy and unhealthy life expectancy differs substantially between women and men among the countries studied. This result highlights differences in health expectancy among relatively homogeneous populations.

Ichiro Tsuji, Catherine Sauvaget, and Shigeru Hisamichi review the results of two recent studies of active life expectancy for older women and men in Japan, finding striking gender differences in the disability process and healthy life expectancy. Drs. Tsuji, Sauvaget, and Hisamichi discuss evolving patterns of education, marriage, and caregiving in Japan, focusing on women, and report on a national long-term care insurance program introduced in Japan in 2000. The policy implications of the active life expectancy results they describe are considered in the context of caregiving and formal long-term care service use and costs.

Sela V. Panapasa's study of Fiji highlights the complexities of defining disability in the context of Fiji and Pacific culture, and prompts us to reconsider the relative ease and simplicity with which the literature often defines disability. Using census and survey data, Dr. Panapasa finds notable gender and socioeconomic differences in healthy life expectancy, and considers the implications of the findings for Fiji and other developing countries. Finally, James N. Laditka and I provide a critical synthesis of the recent active life expectancy literature. Policy implications include a greater understanding of the role of education and racial and ethnic diversity in active life trends, and an increased public policy emphasis on prevention and treatment of chronic disease, together with adoption of more healthy lifestyles.

In sum, the studies in this volume shed new light on variations in healthy life expectancy across groups of older women, as well as differences in life expectancy and active life expectancy between older women and men. Studies examining health expectancies among various groups of older women illustrate the heterogeneity of active life expectancy, and indicate, among other implications, the life cycle effects of poorer health for at-risk populations, defined by income, race, and ethnicity. Results of studies focusing on gender differences highlight differences in diseases and disability onset and progression among older women and men, generally showing that older women live longer both with and without diseases and disability than men. This finding offers challenges and opportunities for practitioners, policymakers, and older women and men and their families. The studies presented in this volume illustrate the broad inquiry addressing health expectancy, and reveal fruitful areas for future research.

REFERENCES

Clendinen, D. (2000). What to call people who used to be old. *New York Times,* July 2: (Section 4) 10.

Colvez, A., & Blanchet, M. (1981). Disability trends in the United States population 1966-76: Analysis of reported causes. *American Journal of Public Health, 71,* 464-471.

Crimmins, E.M., Saito,Y., & Ingegneri, D. (1989). Changes in life expectancy and disability-free life expectancy in the United States. *Population and Development Review, 15,* 235-267.

Davis, W.B., Hayes, C.G., Knowles, M., Riggan, W.B., Van Braggen, J., & Tyroler, H.A. (1985). Geographic variation in declining ischemic heart disease mortality in the United States 1968-1978. 1. Rates and changes, whites, aged 35-74 years. *American Journal of Epidemiology, 122,* 657-672.

Doblhammer, G., & Kytir, J. (2001). Compression or expansion of morbidity? Trends in healthy-life expectancy in the elderly Austrian population between 1978 and 1998. *Social Science & Medicine, 52,* 385-391.

Freedman, V.A., & Martin, L.G. (1998). Understanding trends in functional limitations among older Americans. *American Journal of Public Health, 88,* 1457-1462.

Freudenheim, M. (2001). Decrease in chronic illness bodes well for Medicare costs. *New York Times,* May 8: A4.

Fuchs, V.R. (1974). *Who shall live?* New York: Basic Books.

Hogan, C., Lunney, J., Gabel, J., & Lynn, J. (2001). Medicare beneficiaries' costs of care in the last year of life. *Health Affairs, 20,* 188-195.

Jacobzone, S. (2000). Coping with aging: International challenges. *Health Affairs, 19, 3,* 213-225.

Kinsella, K. (2000). Demographic dimensions of global aging. *Journal of Family Issues, 21,* 542-558.

Lubitz, J., Beebe, J.B., & Baker, C. (1995). Longevity and Medicare expenditures. *New England Journal of Medicine, 332,* 999-1003.

Manton, K.G., Corder, L., & Stallard, E. (1993). Estimates of change in chronic disability and institutional incidence and prevalence rates in the U.S. elderly population from the 1982, 1984, and 1989 National Long Term Care Survey. *Journal of Gerontology: Social Sciences, 48,* S153-S166.

McGovern, P.G., Burke, G.L., Spafka, S.X., Folsom, A.R., & Blackburn, H. (1992). Trends in mortality, morbidity, and risk factor levels for stroke from 1960 through 1990: The Minnesota heart survey. *Journal of the American Medical Association, 268,* 753-759.

Olshansky, S.J., Carnes, B.A., Rogers, R.A., & Smith, L. (1997). Infectious diseases: New and ancient threats to world health. *Population Bulletin, 52,* 1-58.

Olshansky, S.J., & Wilkins, R. (1998). Introduction. *Journal of Aging and Health, 10,* 123-135.

Robine, J.M., Jagger, C., Mathers, C., Crimmins, E., & Suzman, R. (Eds.) (in press). *Determining Health Expectancies.* Baffins Lane, Chichester, Sussex, UK: John Wiley & Sons.

Rowe, J.W., & Kahn, R.L. (1998). *Successful aging.* New York: Pantheon.

U.S. Department of Health, Education, and Welfare (HEW). (1969). *Towards a social report.* Washington, DC: Government Printing Office.

Vita, A.J., Terry, R.B., Hubert, H.B., & Fries, J.F. (1998). Aging, health risks, and cumulative disability. *New England Journal of Medicine, 338,* 1035-1041.

Patterns of Active Life
Among Older Women:
Differences Within and Between Groups

Douglas A. Wolf, PhD
Sarah B. Laditka, PhD
James N. Laditka, DA, MPA

SUMMARY. This study examines the distribution of total, unimpaired, and impaired life for several groups of older women defined by race, education, and marital history. Using data from the 1984-1990 Longitudinal Study of Aging, we model transitions among functional statuses using discrete-time Markov chains, and use microsimulation to produce summary indices of active life. Remaining years of life and the proportion of remaining years with disability vary substantially, both within each group of women studied and between pairs of groups. Of all groups studied, never-married, more-educated white women live the longest, healthiest lives. Ever-married nonwhite women with low education have the shortest life expectancy, and experience the most disability. Our find-

Douglas A. Wolf is Gerald B. Cramer Professor of Aging Studies, Center for Policy Research, Syracuse University, 426 Eggers Hall, Syracuse, NY 13244 (E-mail: DAWolf@maxwell.syr.edu).

Sarah B. Laditka is Associate Professor of Health Services Management and Director of the Center for Health and Aging, State University of New York Institute of Technology.

James N. Laditka is a PhD candidate at the Maxwell School of Citizenship and Public Affairs, and Research Associate of the Center for Policy Research, Syracuse University.

[Haworth co-indexing entry note]: "Patterns of Active Life Among Older Women: Differences Within and Between Groups." Wolf, Douglas A., Sarah B. Laditka, and James N. Laditka. Co-published simultaneously in *Journal of Women & Aging* (The Haworth Press, Inc.) Vol. 14, No. 1/2, 2002, pp. 9-26; and: *Health Expectations for Older Women: International Perspectives* (ed: Sarah B. Laditka) The Haworth Press, Inc., 2002, pp. 9-26. Single or multiple copies of this article are available for a fee from The Haworth Document Delivery Service [1-800-HAWORTH 9:00 a.m. - 5:00 p.m. (EST). E-mail address: getinfo@haworthpressinc.com].

9

ings show that life expectancy is an incomplete indicator of the time women, in particular sub-groups, can expect to live with and without impairment. These findings highlight the heterogeneity of disability processes and life expectancy for older women. *[Article copies available for a fee from The Haworth Document Delivery Service: 1-800-HAWORTH. E-mail address: <getinfo@haworthpressinc.com> Website: <http://www.HaworthPress.com> © 2002 by The Haworth Press, Inc. All rights reserved.]*

KEYWORDS. Active life expectancy, disability, functional status, Markov-chain, microsimulation

INTRODUCTION

As the number of older Americans grows, both public and private institutions face the possibility of increasing demands for health services, accompanied by rising public and private health care costs. Population aging might similarly add to the hidden costs borne by those who provide the most help to older persons, namely family and friends. Public policies often address these informal service providers, as well. For example, many states have instituted caregiver support programs (Feinberg & Pilisuk, 1999), and consequent to the recent reauthorization of the Older Americans Act, the federal government has launched a National Family Caregiver Program (U.S. Department of Health and Human Services, 2001). Planning for the challenges of an aging population can be informed with improved information about patterns of active life. A better understanding of active life patterns among older women is especially important, since women comprise a large majority of our older population. Given their longer lives and more years of disability, women also use more health care than men.

The percentage of United States' households with single adults has increased greatly (Ahlburg & DeVita, 1992; Smeeding, 1999). Blacks have been particularly affected by declining marriage rates and the increase in households headed by women (Taylor, Chatters, Tucker, & Lewis, 1990). Blacks also constitute a growing percentage of the U.S. population (U.S. Bureau of the Census, 1999). In light of these demographic trends, it is important to understand patterns of active life for groups of older women defined by race and marital status.

Research on active life has focused almost exclusively on the *average* number of years an individual can expect to live without, or with, disability, that is on "active" or "inactive" life *expectancy*. Such measures are useful for actuarial calculations. They can be used, for example, to determine the insurance value of long-term care services. But averages have their limitations. At any given age, the likely number of additional years lived with and without disability varies considerably across individuals. This variation occurs within groups defined by characteristics associated with disability processes and longevity; some individuals in the group will experience below-average, and others above-average episodes of disability, and many will never experience disability at all. Between-group differences in averages, and in departures from those averages, occur as well. Thus, when considering broader issues of equity and efficiency in the financing and provision of services, or when targeting programmatic resources, it is useful to recognize the full distribution of active, impaired, and total life, and not only the averages of each. To our knowledge, no past research has explicitly traced the frequency distribution that is implicit in calculations of active life expectancy. Similarly, few previous studies have compared averages of such distributions across groups of older women.

Our study examines variations in three measures commonly reported in the active life expectancy literature: total life, active (unimpaired, or disability free) life, and inactive (impaired, or disabled) life. We examine this variability from two perspectives. First, we show how these measures can vary *within* a given group of older women, where group membership is defined by race, education, and marital status. Second, we investigate differences in total, active, and inactive life expectancy *between* such groups. Our analysis focuses on older women, using data from the 1984 to 1990 Longitudinal Study of Aging (LSOA) and microsimulation techniques.

FACTORS ASSOCIATED WITH DISABILITY AND ACTIVE LIFE EXPECTANCY

Past research has shown that disability prevalence and incidence, and active life expectancy, differ substantially across groups of the older population. Studies have consistently shown that older women with more education live longer and healthier lives than those with less education (Crimmins, Hayward, & Saito, 1996; Crimmins & Saito, 2001; Freedman & Martin, 1999; Land, Guralnik, & Blazer, 1994). Researchers have suggested that education may influence individuals' ability to understand and reduce risk factors, and to adopt healthier life-styles. There is also evidence of notable mortality and morbidity differences between blacks and whites, although findings in this research area are inconsistent. A growing number of researchers have found that white women have both total and active life expectancies greater than those of black women (Crimmins et al., 1996; Crimmins & Saito, 2001; Geronimus, Bound, Waidmann, Colen, & Steffick, 2001; Hayward & Heron, 1999). Researchers point to socioeconomic, cultural, and genetic factors, as well as other advantages and disadvantages across the life span, as likely causes of racial disparities in mortality and morbidity (e.g., Hayward, Crimmins, Miles, & Yang, 2000).

Many studies have examined associations between marital status and mortality. Studies have variously investigated differentials by marital *status,* marital *history,* and marital *events.* For example, Lillard and Waite (1995) modeled mortality risks over a 20-year period for a sample of adults of all ages, finding elevated mortality rates among never-married and separated women (compared to currently-married women), and little difference between the mortality rates of widowed and currently-married women. Lillard and Waite (1995) also found that the benefits of being married grow as the duration of marriage grows. Others have investigated the consequences of experiencing spousal death, or bereavement. Schaefer, Quesenberry, and Wi (1995) found that women's mortality rates were significantly higher 7-12 months after the death of their spouse, but not before or thereafter. Their study did not, however, include comparisons to a never-married group. Korenman, Goldman and Fu (1997), using data from the LSOA, found a significant adverse mortality effect among women widowed more than one year, but not during the first year of widowhood. Their study also failed to find a significant difference between the death rates of currently-married and never-married women, holding several covariates constant.

Goldman, Korenman, and Weinstein (1995) examined the association between marital status and disability, and the mediating role of economic factors in this relationship, using data from the LSOA. They found that never-married women had significantly lower probabilities of being disabled than ever-married women. Including social and economic controls in this research strengthened the relationship between health and marital status. Furthermore, the never-married were the most socially active women (Goldman et al., 1995). These results are consistent with research showing that some unmarried groups create social environments associated with improved health (Anson, 1989), and with other research finding that economic factors explain a large portion of the health differences between married and unmarried women (Hahn, 1993).

The studies on marital status reviewed above consider marital-status differentials in death rates, as well as health or disability prevalence-rate (and in some cases incidence-rate) differences by marital status. None, however, report differences by marital status in active or inactive life expectancy. Differences in total life expectancy associated with marital status *changes* (such as the death of one's spouse) are difficult to compute since the timing of widowhood is itself a random variable. However, results found in Espenshade (1983) allow calculation of remaining total life expectancy (but not active or inactive life expectancy) at age 70, according to marital status at that age. Espenshade's findings indicate that never-married women age 70 can expect to live an additional 14.3 years, while ever-married women can expect to live slightly longer, 14.6 years. Thus, taken together past literature on marital status, health and mortality does not produce unambiguous predictions concerning differences in active and disabled life expectancy by marital status.

DATA AND ANALYTICAL APPROACH

Our study uses data from the 1984, 1986, 1988, and 1990 waves of the Longitudinal Study of Aging. One of the primary objectives of the LSOA was to evaluate changes in functional ability among older individuals in the United States over time. The 1984 baseline survey was administered to a nationally-representative sample of 7,527 non-institutionalized individuals age 70 or older. Those who subsequently entered nursing homes were included in the follow-up interviews. Kovar, Fitti, and Chyba (1992) provide further details about the LSOA. The sample used in this study is restricted to female LSOA respondents whose records contained the information required for our modeling ($n = 4,281$). This sample provided 9,489 instances of functional status transition, from which parameters representing transition probabilities were estimated. Further details regarding sample selection are provided in Laditka and Wolf (1998).

Consistent with previous studies of active life expectancy, an individual's functional status assignment in this study reflects the presence or absence of impairment in the following activities of daily living (ADLs): bathing, eating, dressing, transferring, and using the toilet

(Katz, Ford, Moskowitz, Jackson, & Jaffee, 1963). Individuals were defined as impaired if they reported any difficulty performing one or more of these activities, or if they reported receiving any help carrying out the activity. Previous research provides strong evidence that functional status differs notably between whites and nonwhites, and likelihood-ratio tests confirmed the presence of statistically significant model parameters by race. Thus, we estimated separate models for nonwhite and white women. Nonwhites constituted 8.6% of the sample. Most of the nonwhites (89.7%) were black.

Our models include several covariates representing other factors that have been shown by previous research to be associated with functional status: age, education, and marital status. *Age,* measured in years, appears as a time-varying covariate. *Low Education,* a dichotomous variable, identifies individuals who completed less than 12 years of school (54.7% of the sample). *Ever-married,* also a dichotomous measure, identifies women who had married as of the baseline interview (94.9% of the sample). Our models implicitly assume that no women marry for the first time after age 70, and that educational attainment is fixed as well by age 70.

The model of women's functional-status transitions, the procedure for estimating transition probabilities, and the microsimulation procedure used in this study have been described in detail elsewhere (Laditka & Laditka, 2001; Laditka & Wolf, 1998). Here we use a simpler representation of disability, but more covariates, than in our previous work. Monthly transition probabilities are determined by trinomial logistic regression models. The dependent variables in these models distinguish among three outcomes: transitions to the *unimpaired* (*U*) state (i.e., to having no ADL limitations), to the *impaired* (*I*) state (i.e., having 1-5 ADL limitations), or to *death* (*D*). There is one such multinomial regression equation for persons who begin a month unimpaired, and one for those who begin a month impaired, producing a total of 6 transition probabilities. A total of 16 parameters appear in these two equations, an intercept plus three effect parameters for each of 4 of the functional-status transitions (that is, from either *unimpaired* or *impaired,* to either *impaired* or *death*); the analogous parameters for the 2 transitions to the *unimpaired* state normalized to zero. The estimates were obtained using specialized software designed for this purpose by the authors, written in the SAS IML programming language.

The estimated model parameters were used to compute predicted values of monthly transition probabilities at each age, beginning at age 70, and for every combination of education and ever-married status, separately by race. Those sets of predicted transition probabilities were then used to simulate a large (n = 100,000) sample of individual-level monthly functional-status histories (e.g., sequences such as *U, U, U, U, I, . . . D*) from the month after the 70th birthday until the month of (simulated) death, for each of six groups of women, defined by race, education, and marital status. The percent disabled at age 70 in each microsimulation was chosen to match actual population proportions of older women with the same race, education level, and marital status at ages 70-75 living in the community, through weighted analysis of the 1984 LSOA. Thus, for example, the life course experience of disability was simulated for a population of 100,000 ever-married nonwhite women with high education. In the 1984 LSOA, 6.3% of 70-75-year-olds in this group were disabled (using our definition), so this same proportion of individuals in the simulated population entered the microsimulation disabled. In addition to the six groups for which we conducted simulations, two other groups could be defined by our categories. These two groups were more sparsely represented in the LSOA. Since reliable estimates of the proportion of each group with disability at ages 70-75 were needed to identify starting populations for the microsimulations, these groups were not included in the analysis.

The data produced by the microsimulation procedure were treated as longitudinal survey data and analyzed using standard statistical methods. For example, total life expectancy within the simulated population is simply the average age at death, and unimpaired life expectancy is the average count of months coded "*U*." We investigated the degree of variability in the length of active and inactive life by producing a frequency distribution of the number of years spent in each functional status, and summarize this variability using conventional summary statistics, such as histograms and standard deviations. Because of the very large sizes of the simulated populations, we ignore "sampling" variation in our presentation of results; the means and standard deviations shown are interpreted as population-level values.

RESULTS

Model of Functional Status Transitions

Table 1 shows the estimated coefficients for our model of functional status transitions for whites and nonwhites. For each possible transition, Table 1 presents four coefficients: an intercept and coefficients repre-

TABLE 1. Parameters of Multinomial Logit Models of Functional Status Transitions[a]

	Estimate (SE)[c]	
Origin = U; Destination = I [b]	Whites	Nonwhites
Constant	−5.79 (0.195)***	−4.479 (0.540)***
Age	0.086 (0.006)***	0.051 (0.020)**
Low Education	0.281 (0.069)***	0.052 (0.237)
Ever-Married	−0.037 (0.179)	−0.319 (0.503)
Origin = U; Destination = D [b]		
Constant	−6.674 (0.256)***	−6.445 (1.577)***
Age	0.069 (0.010)***	−0.001 (0.078)
Low Education	−0.040 (0.110)	0.415 (0.651)
Ever-Married	0.008 (0.231)	−0.058 (1.558)
Origin = I; Destination = I [b]		
Constant	3.143 (0.288)***	3.863 (0.777)***
Age	0.034 (0.010)***	0.048 (0.033)
Low Education	−0.045 (0.106)	0.761 (0.386)*
Ever-Married	0.703 (0.245)**	−0.739 (0.737)
Origin = I; Destination = D [b]		
Constant	−2.286 (0.379)***	−2.272 (1.374)
Age	0.091 (0.012)***	0.085 (0.037)*
Low Education	0.039 (0.137)	0.613 (0.488)
Ever-Married	0.815 (0.323)*	0.764 (1.347)

[a]Source: 1984-1990 Longitudinal Study of Aging.
[b]U = Unimpaired; I = Impaired; D = Dead.
[c]SE = Standard Error.
*$p < 0.05$; **$p < 0.01$; ***$p < 0.001$

senting effects of age, education, and marital status. For white women, all of the age coefficients are statistically significant, indicating rising age profiles of relative probabilities of making the indicated transition, relative to the reference category (in each case, a transition to the *unimpaired* state). Among the education effects, only one is significant: women in the low-education group are more likely to become impaired in a given month than are more educated women, other factors being equal. For the white women, the marriage effects are somewhat surprising in view of some past research: ever-married white women are more likely to remain impaired (relative to recovering) and also more likely to die (again, relative to recovering) compared to never-married women. Among nonwhite women, few of the estimated coefficients are statistically significant, although as noted before, global tests indicate that the race-specific sets of regression coefficients are statistically different from each other. For a clearer picture of the within- and between-group patterns of active and disabled life from age 70 onward, we turn to the results of our microsimulations.

Life Course Patterns of Active Life Expectancy

Figures 1 and 2, and Tables 2 and 3 illustrate the main results of our microsimulation analyses. Figure 1 displays frequency distributions for the sample of 100,000 never-married, white women with high education. The Figure shows remaining years of life (top panel), remaining years of unimpaired life (middle panel), and remaining years of impaired life (lower panel). The maximum number of remaining years at age 70 in this group is 48; the maximum of unimpaired years is 11, and of impaired years, 35. Data points at the upper limits of these distributions, attained by only a small number of sample members, are omitted. These frequency distributions illustrate *within* group variability.

The microsimulation results for the women represented by Figure 1 produce a total life expectancy of 14.7 years. These women can expect to live 11.3 of these years without impairment, and the remainder with impairment. For remaining years of life and remaining years of unimpaired life, the histograms of Figure 1 show relatively symmetric, albeit truncated, distributions. The histogram for remaining years of impaired life (bottom panel) is, however, highly skewed, with a substantial percentage of women in the simulated population having zero years of impairment, and only a small percentage living many years impaired. Thus, the within group patterns show that the average number of remaining years, of years spent unimpaired, and particularly of years spent impaired, are poor descriptions of "typical" life experiences for older women: most women's experiences are substantially below (or above) these averages.

The shapes of the corresponding three distributions derived from simulated populations representing other combinations of race, education, and marital status vary somewhat from those in Figure 1. For example, Figure 2 represents the situation of ever-married, nonwhite women. In contrast with the relatively symmetric shape of the histogram in the upper panel of Figure 1, the histogram for remaining years of life in the upper panel of Figure 2 is quite skewed. A comparison of the middle panels of Figures 1 and 2 accentuates the large spike at zero years for nonwhite women; a large number of nonwhite women in this

FIGURE 1. Remaining Years of Unimpaired, Impaired, and Total Life: Never-Married White Women with High Education at Age 70, N = 100,000

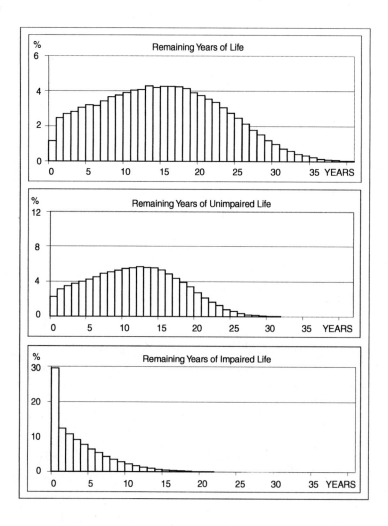

group have *no* remaining full years without impairment beginning at age 70. Further, the distribution of remaining unimpaired years is much more skewed toward fewer years of unimpaired life in Figure 2, again compared with the experience of never-married, highly educated white women represented by Figure 1. Again, we find that life expectancy at

FIGURE 2. Remaining Years of Unimpaired, Impaired, and Total Life: Ever-Married Nonwhite Women with Low Education at Age 70, N = 100,000

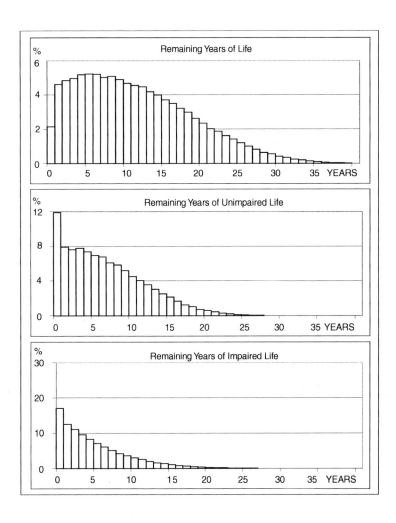

age 70, and also the proportion of life spent both unimpaired and impaired, varies considerably within an otherwise homogeneous group. The distributions, which more accurately characterize the range of experience within a given group, are inadequately portrayed by the averages alone.

TABLE 2. Comparisons of Average Remaining Years of Unimpaired, Impaired, and Total Life by Race, Marital Status, and Education at Age 70[a]

	Group	Age 70 Impairment[b]	Expectancy Type[c]	Mean (SD)[d]
	White		*T*	13.5 (7.6)
(1)	Ever-Married	11.24	*U*	9.6 (6.0)
	High Education		*I*	3.9 (4.3)
	White		*T*	12.7 (7.3)
(2)	Ever-Married	15.86	*U*	8.5 (5.6)
	Low Education		*I*	4.3 (4.3)
	White		*T*	14.7 (8.1)
(3)	Never-Married	4.60	*U*	11.3 (6.2)
	High Education		*I*	3.5 (3.9)
	White		*T*	14.0 (7.9)
(4)	Never-Married	13.06	*U*	10.2 (5.8)
	Low Education		*I*	3.9 (4.0)
	Nonwhite		*T*	13.0 (7.9)
(5)	Ever-Married	6.29	*U*	9.0 (6.0)
	High Education		*I*	4.0 (3.8)
	Nonwhite		*T*	11.2 (7.5)
(6)	Ever-Married	18.22	*U*	6.5 (5.3)
	Low Education		*I*	4.8 (4.7)

[a]Source: 1984-1990 Longitudinal Study of Aging.
[b]Weighted percentage of subgroup at ages 70-75 impaired in 1984 LSOA.
[c]*T* = Total remaining years; *U* = Unimpaired years; *I* = Impaired years.
[d]SD = Standard deviation; means for unimpaired and impaired years may not add to total remaining years due to rounding.

To address both between- and within-group differences, we report in Table 2 the average remaining years of life (i.e., the usual expectancy indicator), average remaining years of unimpaired life, and average remaining years of impaired life, all at age 70, for the six groups of women studied. Table 2 also shows the standard deviations of these variables, a quantitative measure of within-group differences. To highlight between-group differences, we show all possible pairwise com-

TABLE 3. Differences in Life Expectancy in Years for Women at Age 70, by Expectancy Type, for Selected Attributes and Population Subgroups

	Difference in Expectancy by Type		
	Total	Unimpaired	Impaired
Difference between high- and low-education . . .			
white, ever-married	0.8	1.1	−0.4
white, never-married	0.7	1.1	−0.4
nonwhite, ever-married	1.8	2.5	−0.8
Difference between ever- and never-married . . .			
white, low-education	−1.3	−1.7	0.4
white, high-education	−1.2	−1.7	0.4
Difference between white and nonwhite . . .			
ever-married, low-education	1.5	2.0	−0.5
ever-married, high-education	0.5	0.6	−1.0

[a]Source: 1984-1990 Longitudinal Study of Aging

parisons of each expectancy in Table 3, in the form of differences. In Table 3, differences in unimpaired and in impaired years of life sum to the difference in total years of life for each pair of groups considered.

There are a number of interesting findings in Tables 2 and 3. In groups paired across race categories with the same marriage and education characteristics, total life expectancy, and unimpaired life expectancy for whites exceeds that of nonwhites. Nonwhite women can, moreover, expect to spend a smaller proportion of their lives unimpaired than white women. For example, a nonwhite woman with low education who was ever-married (Group 6) can expect to live about 58% of her remaining life unimpaired, while the analogous figure for a white woman with the same characteristics (Group 2) is 67%. More education is associated with somewhat longer life and a smaller proportion of impaired life for ever- or never-married white women, and with a substantially longer life (1.8 years) for nonwhite ever-married women. Interestingly, white women with high education who were never-married live the longest and healthiest lives of all groups studied: whether in the low or high education group, ever-married women's life expectancy is about one and one-third years shorter than otherwise similar never-married women. The apparent advantage of the never-married white women with respect to unimpaired life is even greater (a 1.7 year difference, as shown in Table 3).

Turning to within group differences in life expectancy, we focus on the standard deviation of years remaining in total, unimpaired and impaired life displayed in Table 2. For all groups shown, this measure of within-group variability is considerably larger than any of the between-group differences (in averages) shown in Table 3. In other words, the distributions of total (and of active and inactive) remaining life are centered on different values for different groups, but the distributions overlap to a considerable degree. The ratio of standard deviation to mean (an indicator of *relative* variation) is generally larger for nonwhites than for whites. In addition, the ratio of standard deviation to mean is greater for impaired life, compared with either total remaining years or unimpaired years of life. Finally, in most instances, the standard deviation of impaired life is equal to or greater than its mean. Collectively, these results show that the variability in remaining years of total life, as well as life with and without impairment, is quantitatively substantial.

DISCUSSION

Using a large longitudinal survey of older Americans, we developed a model with which to investigate variability in estimates of total life expectancy, unimpaired life expectancy, and impaired life expectancy for six groups of older women. We found that the variability of total, unimpaired, and impaired life expectancies about their expected (mean) values is substantial. Variability in the pattern of total, unimpaired, and impaired life was revealed by our histograms (Figures 1 and 2) and by the standard deviations obtained for these frequency distributions (Table 2). Most previous research has examined only the average number of years of total, impaired, and unimpaired life. Our findings of substantial, within group variation highlight the uncertainty inherent in forecasting service needs and use, even for specific groups of older people sharing a set of characteristics importantly associated with health and longevity. The highly skewed distributions of impaired life expectancy indicate that relatively small numbers of older women will experience long periods of disability. These findings parallel those for nursing home use (e.g., Murtaugh, Kemper, Spillman, & Carlson, 1997). From a policy perspective, they support policies promoting universal enrollment in long-term care insurance plans to spread the great costs of long-term care across the population.

We also found systematic differences in health expectancies between groups of older women defined by race, education, and marital status. A comparison of histograms for total, active, and inactive life expectancies between groups, exemplified by our comparisons of Figures 1 and 2, illustrated these between group differences qualitatively. Our findings of substantial between-group differences highlight heterogeneity in patterns of active life expectancy for older women. These results provide information that should be useful to those who design or evaluate policies to address disability. They are also relevant to researchers who study the demography of longevity and aging, disability processes, and both formal and informal systems of care for older persons.

Our findings for race and education are consistent with previous studies. We find that nonwhite women, who were primarily blacks in our sample, live shorter, less healthy lives than white women (Hayward & Heron, 1999). Education in our results was positively associated with longer life and better health (Land et al., 1994). Our findings for marital status are of special interest, given recent trends in marriage and family structure toward more households headed by single women. For white women in either education group, the never-married live longer and healthier lives than the ever-married. These results agree with some, but also contradict some, of the mixed findings with respect to marital status, health, disability, and mortality found in past research. Our results are, for example, consistent with research by Goldman et al. (1995), who noted that the LSOA baseline survey excluded individuals in nursing homes–and that the institutionalized are more likely to be unmarried. Goldman et al. (1995) concluded from this observation that the never-married women remaining in the community who participated in the LSOA were likely to have enjoyed better health. Indeed, since the dynamics of institutionalization involve the availability of informal caregivers and the never-married have less access to informal ADL care, it is likely that the never-married remaining in the community enjoyed better health than ever-married community residents. Our results are also consistent with research suggesting that some groups of unmarried women form social relationships associated with better health (Anson, 1989). However, our findings with respect to marital status should be viewed with some caution. Our ever-married group includes currently-married women as well as divorcees and widows. The widowed group undoubtedly contains many recent widows, who, based on past research, can be expected to exhibit temporarily higher-than-expected death rates. Similarly, the currently-married group contains many women who experienced their spouse's death during the follow-up period of data collection, again subjecting them to short-run bereavement effects. The never-married group in our sample is not, in contrast, at risk of such transitory phenomena. Finally, the never-married group constitutes only about 6% of our sample, which renders our results somewhat susceptible to the influence of outliers. Additional research with larger samples and longer follow-up periods could help clarify (and possibly confirm) these patterns.

Our modeling approach allowed us to explore a new dimension in active life expectancy. An important unanswered question is the extent to which our results are specific to the combination of Markovian model specification, estimation technique, and data source used. It should be noted, however, that virtually all past research on active life expectancy relies, either explicitly or implicitly, on a set of assumptions identical to those of our Markovian model. For demographers, our findings about the variability of active life expectancy provide a baseline for more complex models, yet to be developed. They also suggest that research reports of active life expectancy would benefit from more routine analysis of within and between group variability. More information about the full distribution of active and disabled years of life will help identify groups more (or less) likely to be served by social programs, allowing policymakers to better understand complex issues of equity and efficiency.

REFERENCES

Ahlburg, D.A., & DeVita, C.J. (1992). New realities of the American family. *Population Bulletin, 47*, 2-37.

Anson, O. (1989). Marital status and women's health revisited: The importance of a proximate adult. *Journal of Marriage and the Family, 51*, 185-202.

Crimmins, E.M., Hayward, M.D., & Saito, Y. (1996). Differentials in active life expectancy in the older population of the United States. *Journal of Gerontology: Social Sciences, 51B*, S111-S120.

Crimmins, E.M., & Saito,Y. (2001). Trends in healthy life expectancy in the United States, 1970-1999: Gender, racial, and educational differences. *Social Science & Medicine, 52*, 1629-1641.

Espenshade, T.J. (1983). Marriage, divorce, and remarriage from retrospective data: A multiregional approach. *Environment and Planning, Series A, 15*, 1633-1652.

Feinberg, L.F., & Pilisuk, T. (1999). Survey of fifteen states' caregiver support programs: Final report. San Francisco: Family Caregiver Alliance.

Freedman, V.A., & Martin, L.G. (1999). The role of education in explaining and forecasting trends in functional limitations among older Americans. *Demography, 36,* 461-473.

Geronimus, A.T., Bound, J., Waidmann, T.A., Colen, C.G., & Steffick, D. (2001). Inequity in life expectancy, functional status, and active life expectancy across selected black and white populations in the United States. *Demography, 38,* 227-251.

Goldman, N., Korenman, S., & Weinstein, R. (1995). Marital status and health among the elderly. *Social Science and Medicine, 40,* 1717-1730.

Hahn, B.A. (1993) Marital status and women's health: The effect of economic marital acquisitions. *Journal of Marriage and the Family, 55,* 495-504.

Hayward, M.D., Crimmins, E.M., Miles, T.P., & Yang, Y. (2000). The significance of socioeconomic status in explaining the racial gap in chronic health conditions. *American Sociological Review, 65,* 910-930.

Hayward, M.D., & Heron, M. (1999). Racial inequity in active life among adult Americans. *Demography, 36,* 77-91.

Katz, S., Ford, A.B., Moskowitz, R.W., Jackson, B.A., & Jaffee, M.W. (1963). Studies of illness in the aged. The index of ADL: A standardized measure of biological and psychosocial function. *Journal of the American Medical Association, 185,* 914-919.

Korenman, S., Goldman, N., & Fu, H. (1997). Misclassification bias in estimates of bereavement effects. *American Journal of Epidemiology, 145,* 995-1001.

Kovar, M.G., Fitti, J.E., & Chyba, M.M. (1992). *The Longitudinal Study of Aging: 1984-1990.* Vital Health Statistics (28), Hyattsville, MD: National Center for Health Statistics.

Laditka, S.B., & Laditka, J.N. (2001). Effects of improved morbidity rates on active life expectancy and eligibility for long-term care services. *Journal of Applied Gerontology, 20,* 39-56.

Laditka, S.B., & Wolf, D.A. (1998). New methods for analyzing active life expectancy. *Journal of Aging and Health, 10,* 214-241.

Land, K.C., Guralnik, J.M., & Blazer, D.G. (1994). Estimating increment-decrement life tables with multiple covariates from panel data: The case of active life expectancy. *Demography, 31,* 297-319.

Lillard, L.A., & Waite, L.J. (1995). 'Til death do us part: Marital disruption and mortality. *American Journal of Sociology, 100,* 1131-1156.

Murtaugh, C.M., Kemper, P., Spillman, B.C., & Carlson, B.L. (1997). The amount, distribution, and timing of lifetime nursing home use. *Medical Care, 35,* 204-218.

Schaefer, C., Quesenberry, C.P., & Wi, S. (1995). Mortality following conjugal bereavement and the effects of a shared environment. *American Journal of Epidemiology, 141,* 1142-1152.

Smeeding, T.M. (1999). *Social Security reform: Improving benefit adequacy and economic security for women.* Center for Policy Research Aging Studies Program Policy Brief No. 16/1999. Syracuse, NY: Syracuse University.

Taylor, R.J., Chatters, L.M., Tucker, M.B., & Lewis, E. (1990). Developments in research on black families: A decade review. *Journal of Marriage and the Family, 52,* 993-1014.

United States Bureau of the Census. 1999. *Current population reports.* Washington, D.C.

United States Department of Health and Human Services. (2001). HHS launches national family caregiver program. *HHS News,* February 15, 2001 (available on the world-wide web at http://www.aoa.gov/pressroom/pr2001/nlcsplaunch.htm; accessed March 21, 2001).

Health Profiles and Profile-Specific Health Expectancies of Older Women and Men: The Netherlands

Dorly J. H. Deeg, PhD
France Portrait, PhD
Maarten Lindeboom, PhD

SUMMARY. This study focuses on gender differences in health profiles, and examines which health profiles drive gender differences in remaining life expectancy in women and men aged 65 and over in The Netherlands. Data from the first two cycles of the Longitudinal Aging Study Amsterdam (n = 2,141 and 1,659, respectively) were used to calculate health profiles for individuals of 65-85 years. For both women and men, six profiles were found: I. cancer; II. "other" chronic diseases; III. cognitive impairment; IV. frailty or multimorbidity; V. cardiovascular diseases; and VI. good health. The further characterization of these

Dorly J. H. Deeg is affiliated with the Department of Psychiatry and Institute for Research in Extramural Medicine and France Portrait and Maarten Lindeboom are affiliated with the Department of Economics, Vrije Universiteit, Amsterdam, The Netherlands.

The Longitudinal Aging Study Amsterdam is mainly funded by a long-term grant from The Netherlands Ministry of Health, Welfare and Sports.

Address correspondence to: Dorly J. H. Deeg, PhD, Vrije Universiteit / Faculty of Medicine / LASA, Van der Boechorststraat 7, Room H-036, 1081 BT Amsterdam, The Netherlands (E-mail: djh.deeg.emgo@med.vu.nl); (website: http://ssg.scw.vu.nl/lasa/#Deeg).

[Haworth co-indexing entry note]: "Health Profiles and Profile-Specific Health Expectancies of Older Women and Men: The Netherlands." Deeg, Dorly J. H., France Portrait, and Maarten Lindeboom. Co-published simultaneously in *Journal of Women & Aging* (The Haworth Press, Inc.) Vol. 14, No. 1/2, 2002, pp. 27-46; and: *Health Expectations for Older Women: International Perspectives* (ed: Sarah B. Laditka) The Haworth Press, Inc., 2002, pp. 27-46. Single or multiple copies of this article are available for a fee from The Haworth Document Delivery Service [1-800-HAWORTH 9:00 a.m. - 5:00 p.m. (EST). E-mail address: getinfo@haworthpressinc.com].

types showed some gender differences. Remaining life expectancy for women was greater than for men in each health profile. A decomposition into health expectancies showed that both women and men could expect to live about 5 years in good health from age 66. The greatest gender differences in years spent with health problems were found for profile IV and for profile III. Their greater number of years spent in these health states have direct consequences for the type and cost of care women need. *[Article copies available for a fee from The Haworth Document Delivery Service: 1-800-HAWORTH. E-mail address: <getinfo@haworthpressinc.com> Website: <http://www. HaworthPress.com> © 2002 by The Haworth Press, Inc. All rights reserved.]*

KEYWORDS. Health profiles, gender differences, socio-demographics, health expectancy, comorbidity, health care utilization

INTRODUCTION

Like in other developed countries, remaining life expectancy at age 65 has substantially increased in the past century in The Netherlands. Trends since the 1950s, however, show a marked gender difference in gains in life expectancy above age 65 (Van der Kaa, 2000). Whereas during the first half of the twentieth century, the gender difference stayed approximately stable at less than one year (increase from 11.1 to 14.0 years for men and from 11.9 to 14.8 years for women), from 1950 to 1994, the gender difference increased to over four years (increase from 14.0 to 14.8 years for men and from 14.8 to 19.1 in women). The relatively unfavorable development in men is attributed to the rise in cardiovascular diseases and lung cancer, which mainly took place in men (Van Poppel & De Beer, 1996). The increasing gender gap has resulted in an overrepresentation of women in the older population: 70% of all persons aged 80 and over are women.

Comparison of gains in life expectancy with other western European countries shows that the gains in life expectancy at older ages in The Netherlands lag behind, especially due to the slight gains in men (Caselli & Lopez, 1996). It is, however, notable that from the 1980s, the increase in life expectancy in women levels off, whereas the increase in men picks up. This is as true for The Netherlands as it is for several other developed countries (Guralnik et al., 2000). Moreover, in projections for The Netherlands to 2025, life expectancy in men is expected to show faster gains than in women. A large part of this gender difference is attributed to gender difference in smoking trends, and in resulting shifts in lung cancer rates (Valkonen & Van Poppel, 1997; Van Hoorn & De Beer, 1997). The proportion of women among the oldest-age (80+) in 2025 is projected to have shrunk to 61%.

From these demographic data it can be concluded that women constitute the majority of the older population in The Netherlands, but that they face less favorable prospects in terms of life expectancy gains than men. It is important to address the health dynamics that underlie these varying trends.

A well-known paradox exists with respect to gender differences in health in older age: Within age groups, health status is almost invariably better for older men than for older women (e.g., Verbrugge, 1985; Baltes 1998), whereas older women have better chances of survival than older men, given a specific health state (Manton, 1988; Arber & Ginn, 1991). The focus in the present study is on commonly observed sex differences in health status at one point in time and on subsequent short-term survival probability. The questions of interest are how health profiles differ between women and men, and what health profiles drive the gender differences in remaining life expectancy.

METHODS

Sample

LASA is based on a nationally representative cohort, initial ages 55-85 years, with oversampling of men and older-age. The sample was recruited for The Netherlands Stimulating Programme on Research on Aging (NESTOR) study on Living Arrangements and Social Networks of older adults (LSN), which had a response rate of 62.3% (n = 3,805) (Knipscheer et al., 1995). About 10 months after the LSN interview, the participants were approached for the first LASA cycle (1992-93). This cycle is the baseline for the current study (Deeg et al., 1993). Since the purpose of this study is to examine health dynamics of older women and men, and health problems are starting to be more prevalent from age 65, this study is restricted to older persons aged 65-85 years at baseline.

By the start of the LASA baseline, there were 2,553 surviving LSN participants of ages 65-84. Of these survivors, 2,141 subjects took part in the interviews and tests, yielding a response rate of 83.9%; the 16.1% non-response consisted of 4.4% ineligibility through frailty, 1.0% not contacted after eight or more attempts, and 10.7% refusals. Non-response was associated with higher age, but not with sex (Smit & De Vries, 1994).

By the second LASA-cycle (1995-96), 17.8% of baseline participants had died. Of the surviving participants, 94.3% (n = 1,659) were interviewed. Among these participants, a full face-to-face interview and tests were obtained for 83.7%. A short version of the face-to-face interview was completed in 5.3%, a shorter telephone version in 7.3%, and a proxy interview for 3.7% (Smit et al., 1998). The telephone and proxy respondents are not considered in the current study because for them no complete data on health is available.

Data

Because the statistical analyses (Grade of Membership technique, see below) require discrete variables, continuous variables were condensed into categories.

Baseline health. All health data used in this study are gathered at both the first and the second LASA cycle, including self-reported functional limitations, a test of physical performance, self-reported chronic diseases, medical treatment for these diseases, vision, hearing, depressive symptoms, and cognitive impairment.

Functional limitations were indicated by three items: "Can you climb up and down a staircase of 15 steps without stopping?", "Can you cut your own toenails?", and "Can you use your own or public transportation?" Response categories were "yes, without difficulty," "yes, with difficulty," "not able without help," and "cannot" (Van Sonsbeek, 1988; Kriegsman et al., 1997). A "yes, without difficulty" response was scored as 0 and all others as 1. The three items were combined into one score ranging from 0 = having difficulty with none of the three activities through 3 = having difficulty with all three activities.

Upper body performance was measured by asking the respondent to put on and take off a cardigan that was brought in by the interviewer (Magaziner et al., 1997). The time to perform these activities was measured in seconds. Respondents who could not perform the activity were given a score 2; those who could perform the activity were given a score 1 or 0, if the number of seconds needed was above or below the median, respectively.

Cognitive impairments were ascertained using the Dutch translation of the Mini-Mental State Exam (MMSE, Folstein et al., 1975; Launer et al., 1993). On 23 questions and tasks, respondents received one or more points when they gave the correct answer or performed the task correctly. Scores ran from 0 (all answers incorrect) to 30 (unimpaired). Subjects were considered cognitively impaired when their scores were lower than 24 (Tombaugh et al., 1994).

Depressive symptoms were ascertained using the Dutch translation of the 20-item Center for Epidemiologic Studies Depression scale (CES-D, Radloff, 1977; Beekman et al., 1994). Respondents were asked to indicate how often during the past week they had experienced each symptom with response categories 0 = (almost) never to 3 = (almost) always. The score range is 0 (no symptoms) to 60 (maximum number of symptoms). The scale was dichotomized at the generally used cut-off of 16 for a clinically relevant depressive syndrome (Beekman et al., 1997).

Vision and *hearing* were each questioned with two items, indicating difficulty with reading the small print in the paper and with recognizing a face across the room, and difficulty with having a conversation with one person and with a group of four or more persons (Wilson & McNeil, 1981; Van Sonsbeek, 1988). Difficulty with at least one item was coded as 1; no difficulty was coded as 0.

Seven major *chronic disease* categories were questioned in the interview: respiratory diseases, heart diseases, atherosclerosis, diabetes, stroke, arthritis, and cancer. In addition, respondents could indicate whether they had any other chronic somatic condition, for instance hypertension, back problems, or gastro-intestinal disorders. Answers were coded as "no" or "yes." In a validation study, respondents' self-reports were compared to information obtained from their general practitioners, and proved to be reliable (Kriegsman et al., 1996). When a respondent reported a disease, questions were asked regarding the use of prescribed drugs and regular contacts with a physician for this disease. Both questions were combined into a variable "continuing treatment" which is considered as an indicator of medical severity.

Socio-demographic covariates. In addition to gender and age, socio-economic status (indicated by level of education and monthly income), household size, and degree of urbanization were included as measured at baseline.

Socio-economic status was assessed using education (as the highest educational level attained, 1 = less than elementary school, . . . 9 = university), and monthly income from all possible sources. To assess the latter, the respondents were asked to report their income in classes ranging from $417 or less to $2,083 or more. The classes were converted to the median income. If the respondent had a partner, the partner's income was also asked. In this case, a correction factor of 0.7 was applied to obtain an adjusted adult equivalent (Schiepers, 1988). Four income classes were then constructed: less than or equal to $730 (the Dutch minimum wage in 1993), $731-$1,042, $1,043-$1,667, and $1,668 or higher. Because missing values in the income variable were more frequent (15%) than in other variables, they were imputed on the basis of a non-linear regression model of income on other socio-demographic variables.

Other socio-demographic variables were type of household (0 = living with others, 1 = living alone), and degree of urbanization of the municipality where the respondent lived (1 = rural, . . . 9 = highly urban).

Statistical Analyses

The Grade of Membership method (GoM) is a flexible, non-parametric method, designed to calculate health profiles representing type and degree of health disorders (Manton & Woodbury, 1982; Manton et al., 1992). GoM identifies simultaneously latent, multidimensional profiles ("pure types"), as well as the degree to which sample members fit into these profiles. The pure types are not necessarily represented by individual sample members. The degree of similarity between pure types and respondents ("grades of membership") are described by weights that have values between 0 and 1, and that sum to 1 over all profiles. The GoM approach allows for different degrees of impairment among individuals, as well as for comorbidity, i.e., the occurrence of various health problems at the same time. Both aspects are important when considering the health status of older persons. First, health status is best considered as a continuum, rather than as a dichotomy (McKinley, 1995). Second, comorbidity is widely prevalent among older persons (Schellevis et al., 1993).

The grades of membership obtained were used in subsequent modeling of joint health status and mortality. The two cycles of longitudinal data collection are used in order to take into account unobserved, time-invariant individual effects (e.g., genetic factors), which are expected to play a role in the determination of health status. However, when using two cycles, attrition has to be dealt with, as this is likely to be associated with health status, the main focus of this study. Preliminary analyses showed that attrition due to mortality (17.8% of initial participants, and 79.1% of total attrition) is clearly associated with initial health status. Attrition due to mortality is taken into account by augmenting the statistical model with an equation predicting between-cycle mortality, which is estimated jointly with the equations predicting health status for the two cycles (Portrait et al., 2000a). Respondents who dropped out for other reasons than mortality are a mixed group in terms of health status, and are omitted from the analyses.

A first step in the analysis is the calculation of pure types and grades of membership for women and men separately, to evaluate possible gender differences between health profiles. In a second step, parameter estimates for the joint model of health status, mortality, and socio-demographic characteristics are calculated for each gender. Third, based on the pooled data of women and men, gender-, age-, and profile-specific mortality probabilities are calculated. These probabilities are used to calculate profile-specific remaining life expectancies from age 65 for each gender. Because the interval between two cycles is three years, the calculation of the remaining life expectancy is based on successive three-year age groups. The mid-year of the first age group (65-67 years) is 66. Therefore, the remaining life expectancies actually calculated are from age 66 onward. In a last step, health expectancies are calculated for a person of "average" health by decomposing the average remaining life expectancy according to the profiles.

RESULTS

Characterization of Health Profiles

For both women and men, the GoM analyses yielded six pure types (Table 1). Addition of a seventh pure type to the model did not result in a significantly improved likelihood function. The probability profiles of the 22 health indicators in each pure type are compared to the sample frequencies of the health indicators to characterize the types.

From the frequencies of the 22 health indicators, it is readily seen that both the physical and the mental health status of women was worse as compared to men. For example, only 39% of women had no functional limitations, versus 58% of men, and 79% of women had no clinically relevant depressive symptoms, versus 88% of men. Among the chronic diseases, 50% of women reported arthritis, versus 26% of men, and 39% of women reported other diseases, versus 29% of men. On the other hand, women reported heart diseases less often than men: 19% versus 28%, and 56% of women performed well on the upper body test versus 37% of men.

These differences in frequencies of health problems, however, did not lead to very different health profiles for women and men. The following "pure types" were found:

TABLE 1. Health Profiles Obtained from Grade of Membership Analysis, Longitudinal Aging Study Amsterdam, First Cycle (1992-93)

a. Females

	Score	Frequency	Health Profile (Pure Type)					
			I. Canc	II. Other	III. Cogn	IV. Frail	V. CVD	VI. Good
Functional limitations	0	0.39	0.00	0.57	0.00	0.00	0.05	1.00
	1	0.23	0.00	0.43	1.00	0.00	0.36	0.00
	2	0.18	1.00	0.00	0.00	0.01	0.41	0.00
Upper body performance	0	0.56	0.47	0.67	0.62	0.25	0.46	0.69
	1	0.41	0.52	0.33	0.37	0.67	0.54	0.31
Cognitive impairment	0	0.85	0.82	1.00	0.61	0.65	1.00	1.00
Depressive syndrome	0	0.79	1.00	0.87	1.00	0.34	0.87	1.00
Vision problems	0	0.82	1.00	0.86	1.00	0.46	0.90	1.00
Hearing problems	0	0.92	1.00	1.00	1.00	0.76	0.96	1.00
COPD	0	0.88	1.00	1.00	1.00	0.74	0.75	1.00
Treatment COPD	0	0.91	1.00	1.00	1.00	0.80	0.83	1.00
Heart disease	0	0.81	1.00	1.00	1.00	1.00	0.00	1.00
Treatment heart disease	0	0.83	1.00	1.00	1.00	1.00	0.00	1.00
Atherosclerosis	0	0.89	0.95	1.00	1.00	0.76	0.71	1.00
Treatment atherosclerosis	0	0.92	1.00	1.00	1.00	0.80	0.86	1.00
Diabetes	0	0.89	1.00	1.00	1.00	0.67	0.96	1.00
Treatment diabetes	0	0.90	1.00	1.00	1.00	0.68	1.00	1.00
Stroke	0	0.94	1.00	1.00	1.00	0.87	0.87	1.00
Treatment stroke	0	0.96	1.00	1.00	1.00	0.90	0.89	1.00
Arthritis	0	0.50	0.00	0.87	0.00	0.59	0.59	1.00
Treatment arthritis	0	0.77	0.77	1.00	0.77	0.31	1.00	1.00
Cancer	0	0.87	0.55	1.00	1.00	0.80	1.00	1.00
Treatment cancer	0	0.92	0.77	1.00	1.00	0.88	1.00	1.00
Other chronic diseases	0	0.61	1.00	0.00	1.00	0.13	1.00	1.00
Treatment other diseases	0	0.29	1.00	0.00	1.00	0.47	1.00	1.00

b. Males

	Score	Frequency	I. Canc	II. Other	III. Cogn	IV. Frail	V. CVD	VI. Good
Functional limitations	0	0.58	0.46	0.86	0.00	0.00	1.00	1.00
	1	0.21	0.00	0.00	1.00	0.28	0.00	0.00
	2	0.11	0.38	0.14	0.00	0.30	0.00	0.00
Upper body performance	0	0.37	0.42	0.40	0.04	0.12	0.58	0.55
	1	0.60	0.58	0.58	0.93	0.80	0.42	0.44
Cognitive impairment	0	0.88	1.00	0.93	0.73	0.76	0.96	1.00
Depressive syndrome	0	0.88	0.85	1.00	0.91	0.64	1.00	1.00
Vision problems	0	0.89	0.94	0.88	0.94	0.70	1.00	1.00
Hearing problems	0	0.92	1.00	1.00	0.84	0.80	1.00	1.00
COPD	0	0.84	0.83	1.00	0.95	0.60	1.00	1.00
Treatment COPD	0	0.88	0.89	1.00	1.00	0.67	1.00	1.00
Heart disease	0	0.72	1.00	1.00	1.00	0.30	0.17	1.00
Treatment heart disease	0	0.76	1.00	1.00	1.00	0.40	0.16	1.00
Atherosclerosis	0	0.88	1.00	1.00	1.00	0.62	0.88	1.00
Treatment atherosclerosis	0	0.91	1.00	1.00	1.00	0.70	0.91	1.00
Diabetes	0	0.91	1.00	1.00	1.00	0.71	1.00	1.00
Treatment diabetes	0	0.91	1.00	1.00	1.00	0.72	1.00	1.00
Stroke	0	0.91	1.00	1.00	1.00	0.71	1.00	1.00
Treatment stroke	0	0.93	1.00	1.00	1.00	0.79	1.00	1.00
Arthritis	0	0.74	0.65	0.82	0.61	0.44	1.00	1.00
Treatment arthritis	0	0.90	0.91	1.00	0.91	0.73	1.00	1.00
Cancer	0	0.91	0.78	0.97	1.00	0.82	1.00	1.00
Treatment cancer	0	0.96	0.88	0.97	1.00	0.84	1.00	1.00
Other chronic diseases	0	0.71	1.00	0.00	1.00	0.57	1.00	1.00
Treatment other diseases	0	0.81	1.00	0.00	1.00	0.92	1.00	1.00

I. Cancer and mild arthritis;
II. Severe "other" chronic diseases, few functional limitations;
III. Cognitive impairment and mild arthritis;
IV. Frailty, including severe arthritis, chronic obstructive pulmonary diseases (COPD), atherosclerosis, stroke, diabetes, mild cancer, mild "other" chronic diseases, cognitive impairment, depressive symptoms, vision and hearing problems;
V. Cardiovascular diseases;
VI. Good health.

Although these descriptions of the health profiles are valid for both genders, within the profiles there were some gender differences. Pure type I was further characterized by functional limitations, but for women to a lesser extent than for men. Men in pure type I had relatively many depressive symptoms (probability 0.15 versus sample frequency 0.12); women were relatively often cognitively impaired (probability 0.15 versus sample frequency 0.12). Pure type II was further characterized by depressive symptoms in women, but not in men. Men in pure type III more often had a poor upper body performance than women in this pure type. Men in pure type IV were also likely to have heart disease; women in this frail pure type were not. Finally, whereas pure type V for men was characterized by heart diseases only, women in this pure type in addition had functional limitations, poor upper body performance, COPD, atherosclerosis, and stroke. The characterizations for men and women were tested against the null hypothesis of no difference using a likelihood ratio test in which the likelihood function of the model for males and females combined was compared with the sum of the likelihood functions of the models for males and females separately. The test result was significant, indicating that the probability profiles differed for men and women. However, these differences stem from gender differences within the health profiles and not between the health profiles. Therefore, they do not affect the general characterization of the pure types.

The average grades of membership of women and men in each health profile correspond to the prevalences in the population (Table 2). Pure type VI (good health) is the most prevalent. However, relatively few women as compared to men are characterized by this profile (0.27 vs. 0.38). A profile that is almost equally prevalent in women, but less frequent in men, is pure type IV (frailty): 0.24 vs. 0.18 in men. Pure types I (cancer) and II (other diseases) are also relatively prevalent in women: 0.12 vs. 0.08 (cancer) and 0.16 vs. 0.12 (other diseases) in men. By contrast, pure type V (cardiovascular diseases) is relatively prevalent in men (0.16 vs. 0.09 in women).

Correlates of Health Profiles

A further characterization of the six health profiles is achieved by including socio-demographic covariates in a joint model of mortality and five of the six pure types. The sixth pure type, good health, is omitted to avoid redundancy. In Table 3, higher coefficients are associated with a greater likelihood of mortality or a greater grade of membership in the pure types. Statistical significance is tested using the Student T-test, with a critical value of 1.96.

Of the five health profiles, type IV (frailty) shows the greatest association with mortality. In the joint model, other health profiles do not add to the explanation of mortality. Of the socio-demographic covariates, age has the most pervasive effect: higher age is associated with both mortality and all health profiles except for type II (other diseases). Education is not associated with mortality, nor with pure types I (cancer), II (other diseases), and III (cognitive impairments). However, lower education is associated with a higher grade of membership in type IV (frailty), and in type V (cardiovascular diseases). The strengths of these associations differ between genders: with frailty it is significant only in women, and with cardiovascular diseases it is significant only in men. Income shows two associations only in men: a lower income is associated with greater mortality and with a higher grade of membership in type I (cancer). Living alone is associated with types IV (frailty) and V (cardiovascular diseases). Again, the association is significant only in men. Moreover, the two associations have opposite directions: men living alone are more likely to have cardiovascular diseases; men living with others are more likely to be frail. Finally, degree of urbanization is

TABLE 2. Average Grade of Membership of Women and Men in the Six Health Profiles

	Females	Males
Type I. Cancer	0.12	0.08
Type II. Other diseases	0.16	0.12
Type III. Cognitive impairments	0.11	0.09
Type IV. Frailty	0.24	0.18
Type V. Cardiovascular diseases	0.09	0.16
Type VI. Good health	0.27	0.38

TABLE 3. Socio-Demographic Covariates of Mortality (1992-93/1995-96) and Grades of Membership in Five Health Profiles

		Females		Males	
		Coefficient	T-test	Coefficient	T-test
Mortality	I. Cancer	0.13	0.38	0.23	0.76
	II. Other	−0.17	−0.61	0.04	0.14
	III. Cognitive	−0.14	−0.44	0.09	0.34
	IV. Frail	*1.32*	*3.79*	*1.55*	*5.48*
	V. CVD	0.45	1.35	0.52	1.79
	Age	*5.04*	*−6.87*	*4.65*	*5.06*
	Education	−0.27	−0.83	−0.22	−0.84
	Income	−0.23	−0.74	*−0.64*	*−2.12*
	Living alone	0.15	1.13	0.11	0.84
	Urbanization	−0.02	−0.09	−0.01	−0.05
	Constant	*−5.72*	*−6.87*	−4.75	−0.56
Type I. Cancer	Age	*0.60*	*5.50*	*0.55*	*4.42*
	Education	0.04	1.20	−0.08	−1.85
	Income	0.06	1.40	*−0.20*	*−4.21*
	Living alone	−0.01	−0.73	−0.03	−1.16
	Urbanization	−0.02	−0.71	*0.10*	*3.54*
	Constant	*−0.49*	*−4.75*	*−0.42*	*−3.49*
Type II. Other	Age	−0.26	−1.43	0.20	1.06
	Education	−0.02	−0.30	0.06	0.97
	Income	−0.01	−0.20	0.02	0.30
	Living alone	−0.02	−0.67	−0.02	−0.45
	Urbanization	*−0.07*	*−2.03*	−0.01	−0.31
	Constant	0.25	1.47	−0.31	−1.66
Type III. Cognitive	Age	*0.54*	*3.83*	*0.65*	*4.38*
	Education	−0.05	−1.00	−0.04	−0.74
	Income	−0.02	−0.34	0.02	0.41
	Living alone	0.03	1.26	0.00	0.09
	Urbanization	*−0.10*	*−3.28*	0.05	1.45
	Constant	*−0.37*	*−2.89*	*−0.66*	*−4.55*
Type IV. Frail	Age	1.36	9.32	*1.41*	*9.18*
	Education	*−0.13*	*−5.03*	−0.06	−1.26
	Income	−0.07	−1.54	−0.04	−0.79
	Living alone	−0.01	−0.61	*−0.08*	*−3.38*
	Urbanization	0.03	1.11	*0.07*	*2.23*
	Constant	*−0.91*	*−6.83*	−1.11	−7.53
Type V. CVD	Age	*0.70*	*5.31*	*0.94*	*5.36*
	Education	−0.07	−1.63	*−0.12*	*−2.27*
	Income	−0.04	−1.02	0.10	1.70
	Living alone	−0.01	−0.26	*0.12*	*4.21*
	Urbanization	0.04	1.30	0.06	1.54
	Constant	*−0.62*	*−5.06*	*−0.97*	*−5.65*

Note: Numbers in italics are statistically significant at p < 0.05

associated with all health profiles except cardiovascular diseases (type V). However, the strengths of the associations differ between genders. In men, living in a highly urban area is associated with a higher grade of membership in types I (cancer) and IV (frailty). In women these associations are not significant. On the other hand, women living in a more rural area have higher grades of membership in types II (other diseases) and III (cognitive impairments).

It can be summarized that there are not only gender differences in the characterization of the health profiles, but also in the socio-demographic covariates that further characterize the health profiles.

Remaining Life Expectancies

The calculations of the remaining life expectancies of women and men at age 66 are based on the six pure types as obtained in the full sample including both genders for two reasons. First, the general characterization of the pure types did not differ between the genders. Second, the purpose is to examine which health profiles drive the gender differences in survival. This research question requires a comparison of remaining life expectancies that is based on the same health profiles in women and men.

The average remaining life expectancies at age 66 for females and males are 17.7 and 12.7 years, respectively (Table 4, left part). These correspond well with the remaining life expectancies for the total Dutch population at age 66 in 1993: 17.4 and 13.0, respectively (NCBS, 1995). Considering specific health profiles, it should be noted that these remaining life expectancies are calculated based on the assumption that individuals remain in the pure type that they are in at age 66. This assumption is not realistic, but serves to make a maximal distinction between the pure types in terms of remaining life expectancy. Not surprisingly, the good health profile has the longest remaining life expectancy. The pure type frailty (type IV) has the shortest life expectancy at age 66 for both women and men: 7.6 and 4.2 years, respectively. One other pure type, cardiovascular diseases (type V), also has a relatively short life expectancy for both women and men: 16.2 and 11.0 years, respectively. All other pure types have remaining life expectancies that are relatively long as compared to 66-year-olds with an average health status. Interestingly, women in pure types II (other chronic diseases) and III (cognitive impairments) have greater remaining life expectancies than women in the pure type good health (type VI): 23.6, 23.4, and 21.7 years, respectively. Males in pure type VI do have the longest re-

TABLE 4. Remaining Life Expectancy at Age 66 in Six Health Profiles, and Decomposition of Remaining Life Expectancy at Age 66 in Each Health Profile for "Average" Health Status

| | Total life expectancy | | Decomposed life expectancy | |
	Females	Males	Females	Males
Average health status			18.4	11.5
Type I. Cancer	20.2	14.0	2.2	0.9
Type II. Other diseases	23.6	16.4	2.9	1.3
Type III. Cognitive impairments	23.4	15.7	2.1	1.0
Type IV. Frailty	7.7	4.2	4.4	2.0
Type V. Cardiovascular diseases	16.2	11.0	1.6	1.8
Type VI. Good health	21.7	16.9	5.0	4.4

maining life expectancy (16.7 years), but the difference with pure types II and III is very small: 16.4 and 15.7 years, respectively. The remaining life expectancy in pure type I (cancer) is closer to average for both genders: 20.2 and 14.0 for females and males, respectively.

Another way to distinguish between pure types is to postulate a person of average health status at age 66, and to calculate the number of years to be spent in each pure type relative to the total remaining life expectancy. This calculation is based on the average of the grades of membership in the pure types for each gender-age combination. Women are thus expected to spend 5.0 years in good health (type VI), which compares to 4.4 years in men (table 4, right part). The next largest number of years is spent in frailty (type IV): 4.4 years for women and 2.0 years for men. The expected life time spent in the other types are shorter, and show more divergence between women and men. Women can be expected to spend a relatively longer period in pure types II (other diseases), I (cancer), and III (cognitive impairments) than men, but a relatively shorter period in pure type V (cardiovascular diseases).

DISCUSSION

In the older population of The Netherlands, clear gender differences in level of health were found. Generally, women were impaired more often and in more respects than men. These differences proved to be mainly quantitative; the six health profiles that were determined did not differ substantially between the genders. We did find slight variations within the health profiles of women and men in terms of comorbidity and physical limitations. Women generally had more limitations, except in the cognitively impaired profile, in which men had more upper body limitations. Most notably, in the heart disease profile, women were not only more limited than men, but also had substantial comorbidity. Men in this profile, however, had no comorbidity. By contrast, the frail profile for men was characterized by comorbidity of all chronic diseases, whereas for women heart disease was absent from the frail profile. These differences can be interpreted that, once started, a disease in women follows a longer and more severe course with a greater likelihood of concurrent diseases, than in men.

Evidently, the health profiles obtained partly depend on the initial selection of the health indicators in terms of specificity and coverage of health status aspects. The findings from the present study can be roughly compared to the findings based on a study in a representative sample of the U.S. population (Manton et al., 1992). Despite the fact that they include neither direct indicators of chronic diseases nor mental health indicators, Manton and colleagues (1992) report the same number of health dimensions as were found in the present study, with very similar characterization. Furthermore, gender differences within the health profiles may be partly attributable to characteristics of the health indicators used. In particular, this may be true for upper body limitations. These were measured using a cardigan test. Dutch men are less accustomed to wearing a cardigan than women, and thus may be slower in putting it on and off. It is, therefore, possible that the observed limitations in cognitively impaired men are not so much an expression of decreased physical ability, but instead an additional manifestation of their cognitive impairment.

A further characterization of the health profiles using socio-demographic variables demonstrated several gender differences. Education was associated with frailty in women, but not in men; by contrast, education was associated with cardiovascular diseases in men but not in women. In addition, income was associated with morbidity (i.e., cancer) only in men. Note that frailty in women encompassed multimorbidity but no cardiovascular diseases, whereas in men it encompassed multimorbidity of all diseases. These findings suggest that in the older population of The Netherlands, socio-economic health differences are of a different nature for each gender. First, socio-economic differences in cardiovascular diseases are prominent in men as opposed to women. This finding is replicated in other European countries (Kåreholt, 2001). Second, socio-economic health differences in women are based on non-cardiovascular health problems that occur frequently in old age. This finding may explain why studies in younger populations have found weaker associations between education and morbidity in women than in men (Cavelaars et al., 1998).

Of the other socio-demographic variables, living alone was associated with two health profiles in men only. Men living alone had a greater probability of having cardiovascular diseases, which corresponds to the greater marital status differential with respect to general morbidity and mortality in men as compared to women, as well as the greater risk of heart diseases in unmarried versus married men reported in earlier studies (Samuelsson & Dehlin, 1993; Joung et al., 1996; Malcolm & Dobson, 1989). By contrast, men living with others had a greater probability of being frail. Possibly, these older men have moved in with others because of their deteriorating health, and men living alone were able to do so because they were not frail (Pignatti et al., 2000). Finally, men in urban areas were more likely to have cancer or to be frail, whereas women in rural areas were more likely to have other chronic diseases and cognitive impairments. The finding with respect to men fits in with evidence from other studies on the unfavorable effects of an urban environment on health in general, and particularly on (lung) cancer (Verheij, 1996). The finding with respect to women fits in with the weak, but favorable effect of a rural versus an urban environment on general health that has been reported earlier (Krout, 1989). It must, however, be kept in mind that the health profiles that do show differences in women are characterized by a relatively mild morbidity. These findings emphasize the usefulness of considering specific health profiles rather than general health problems when describing gender differences in health.

The gender differences between the health profiles with respect to both average grade of membership and remaining life time are especially pertinent to health care planning and costs. A first observation was that fewer women than men are in good health, but these fewer women live longer if they stay in this state. Second, women are more likely to be frail, have cancer, have other diseases, and be cognitively impaired than men. Note that arthritis is included in the health profiles that are mainly characterized by frailty, cancer, and cognitive impairment. In numerous publications, arthritis has been shown to be more prevalent in women than in men (Fried & Bush, 1988). The greater risk of cognitive impairment in women corresponds to the findings from a cross-European study, which specified that this increased risk is limited to Alzheimer's disease but does not extend to vascular dementia

(Andersen et al., 1999). In all health profiles where women are predominant, women have longer remaining life expectancies. Especially, cognitive impairment requires intensive long-term care (Meerding et al., 1998; Portrait et al., 2000b). The fact that this care is needed during a long period of remaining life time, makes it extra costly. Third, men more often have cardiovascular diseases than women, but women have a longer remaining life expectancy in this profile. Moreover, the sex specific grade of membership analysis showed that women in this profile more often have comorbidity and mobility impairments than men. The finding of greater comorbidity is supported by evidence from clinical studies in both the U.S. and Europe (Coronado et al., 1997; Herman et al., 1997). As these comorbid impairments are associated with high health care costs, and cardiovascular diseases in themselves are care-intensive (Meerding et al., 1998; Portrait et al., 2000b), again this increases the cost of care for older women.

It has been projected that the proportion of the older population will rise with 43% between 1995 and 2015 in The Netherlands (Verkleij & Mackenbach, 1998). Our data highlight that in an aging society like the Netherlands, health care costs are likely to increase. Moreover, the need for care services will be increasingly greater than cure facilities (Meerding et al., 1998). Therefore, it is important that the proportion of older persons in the care-intensive health profiles will be reduced. This is possible, in principle, by improving the means for prevention and treatment. Improvements in health status, however, have been shown to lead to smaller reductions in use of long-term services in women than in men (Laditka & Laditka, 2001). The health of older women might benefit from the development of gender-specific risk interventions (Wenger, 1998). The gender-specific knowledge base for such interventions and their effects on need for care is still lacking. The study presented here shows that it is particularly urgent to expand our knowledge base pertaining to gender-specific prevention and treatment of cognitive impairments, arthritis, and cardiovascular diseases.

A final note concerns the decreases in gender differences in older-age mortality that have been noted in The Netherlands as well as in several other developed countries. Since these decreases are attributed to life style factors such as smoking, which increases the risk of chronic diseases such as cancer and cardiovascular diseases, it is likely that the observed gender differences in health profiles are subject to change in the near future. Therefore, it will be necessary to repeatedly update the health profiles and to examine time trends in profile-specific health expectancies for women and men.

REFERENCES

Andersen, K., Anderson, K., Launer, L.J., Dewey, M.E., Letenneur, L., Ott, A., Copeland, J.R.M., Dartigues, J.F., Kragh-Sorensen, P., Baldereschi, M., Brayne, C., Lobo, A., Martinez-Lage, J.M., Stijnen, & T., Hofman, A. (1999). Gender differences in the incidence of AD and vascular dementia: The EURODEM Studies. *Neurology 53*, 1992-1997.

Arber, S., & Ginn, J. (1991). Gender, class, and health in later life. In: S. Arber, J. Ginn (Eds.). *Gender and later life. A sociological analysis of resources and constraints.* Sage Publications, London, pp. 107-128.

Baltes, M.M., Freund, A.M., & Horgas, A.L. (1998). Men and women in the Berlin Aging Study. In P.B. Baltes, & K.U. Mayer (Eds.). *The Berlin Aging Study, Aging from 70 to 100.* Cambridge University Press, Cambridge, pp. 259-281.

Beekman, A.T.F., Deeg, D.J.H., Van Limbeek, J., Braam, A.W., De Vries, M.Z., & Van Tilburg, W. (1997). Criterion validity of the Center for Epidemiologic Studies Depression scale (CES-D): Results from a community based sample of older subjects in the Netherlands. *Psychological Medicine 27*, 231-235.

Beekman, A.T.F., Van Limbeek, J., Deeg, D.J.H., Van Tilburg, W., & Wouters, L (1994). Een screeningsinstrument voor depressie bij Nederlandse ouderen in de algemene bevolking: De bruikbaarheid van de Center for Epidemiologic Studies Depression Scale (CES-D) [Screening for depression in the elderly in the community: Using the Center for Epidemiologic Studies Depression Scale (CES-D) in the Netherlands]. Tijdschrift voor Gerontologie en Geriatrie 25, 95-103. In Dutch.

Caselli, G., & Lopez, A.D. (Eds.) (1996). *Health and mortality among elderly populations.* Oxford: Clarendon Press.

Cavelaars, A.E.J.M., Kunst, A.E., Geurts, J.J.M., Crialesi, R., Grötvedt, L., Helmert, U., Lahelma, E., Lundberg, O., Matheson, J., Mielck, A., Mizrahi, A., Mizrahi, A., Rasmussen, N.K., Regidor, E., Spuhler, T., & Mackenbach, J.P. (1998). Differences in self reported morbidity by educational level: A comparison of 11 Western European countries. *Journal of Epidemiology and Community Health 52*, 219-227.

Coronado, B.E., Griffith, J.L., Beshansky, J.R., & Selker, H.P. (1997). Hospital mortality in women and men with acute cardiac ischemia: A prospective multicenter study. *Journal of the American College of Cardiology 29*, 1490-1496.

Deeg, D.J.H., Knipscheer, C.P.M., & Van Tilburg, W. (Eds.) (1993). Autonomy and well-being in the aging population: Concepts and design of the Longitudinal Aging Study Amsterdam. NIG Trendstudies no. 7. Bunnik: Netherlands Institute of Gerontology, 1993.

Folstein, M.F., Folstein, S.E., & McHugh, P.R. (1975). "Mini-Mental State": A practical method for grading the cognitive state of patients for the clinician. *Journal of Psychiatric Research* 12, 89-198.

Fried, L., & Bush, T. (1988). Morbidity as a focus of preventive health care in the elderly. *Epidemiological Review* 10, 48-64.

Guralnik, J.M., Balfour, J.L., & Volpato, S. (2000). The ratio of older women to men: Historical perspectives and cross-national comparisons. *Aging: Clinical and Experimental Research 12*, 65-76.

Herman, B., Greiser, E., & Pohlabeln, H. (1997). A sex difference in short-term survival after initial acute myocardial infarction: The MONICA-Bremen Acute Myocardial Infarction Register, 1985-1990. *European Heart Journal* 18, 963-970.

Joung, I.M.A., Glerum, J.J., Kardaun, J.W.P.F., & Mackenbach, J.P. (1996). The contribution of specific causes of death to mortality differences by marital status in the Netherlands. *European Journal of Public Health* 6, 142-149.

Kåreholt, I. (2001). The relationship between heart problems and mortality in different social classes. *Social Science and Medicine* 52, 1391-1402.

Knipscheer, C.P.M., De Jong Gierveld, J., Van Tilburg, T.G., & Dykstra, P.A. (Eds.) (1995). *Living arrangements and social networks of older adults.* Amsterdam: VU University Press.

Kriegsman, D.M.W., Deeg, D.J.H., Van Eijk, J.T.M., Penninx, B.W.J.H., & Boeke, A.J.P. (1997). Do disease specific characteristics add to the explanation of mobility limitations in patients with different chronic diseases? A study in the Netherlands. *Journal of Epidemiology and Community Health* 51, 676-685.

Kriegsman, D.M.W., Penninx, B.W.J.H., Van Eijk, J.T.M., Boeke, A.J.P., & Deeg, D.J.H. (1996). Self-reports and general practitioner information on the presence of chronic diseases in community-dwelling elderly. A study on the accuracy of patients' self-reports and on determinants of inaccuracy. *Journal of Clinical Epidemiology* 49, 1407-1417.

Krout, J.A. (1989). Rural versus urban differences in health dependence among the elderly population. *International Journal of Aging and Human Development* 28, 141-156.

Laditka, S.B., & Laditka, J.N. (2001). Effects of improved morbidity rates on active life expectancy and eligibility for long-term care services. *Journal of Applied Gerontology* 20, 39-56.

Launer, L.J., Dinkgreve, M.H.A.M., Jonker, C., Hooijer, C., & Lindeboom, J. (1993). Are age and education independent correlates of the Mini-Mental State Exam performance of community-dwelling elderly? *Journal of Gerontology: Psychological Sciences* 48, 271-277.

Magaziner, J., Zimmerman, S.I., Gruber-Baldini, A.L., Hebel, J.R., & Fox, K.M. (1997). Proxy reporting in five areas of functional status. Comparison with self-reports and observations of performance. *American Journal of Epidemiology* 146, 418-428.

Malcolm, J.A., & Dobson, A.J. (1989). Marriage is associated with a lower risk of ischaemic heart disease in men. *Medical Journal of Australia* 151, 185-188.

Manton, K.G. (1988). A longitudinal study of functional change and mortality in the United States. *Journal of Gerontology* 43 (Suppl 5), S153-S161.

Manton, K.G., & Woodbury, M.A. (1982). A new procedure for analysis of medical classification. *Methods of Information in Medicine* 21, 210-220.

Manton, K.G., Woodbury, M.A., Stallard, E., & Corder, L.S. (1992). The use of grade of membership techniques to estimate regression relationships. *Sociological Methodology* 10, 321-379.

McKinley, J.B. (1995). The new public health approach to improving physical activity and autonomy in older populations. In E. Heikkinen, J. Kuusinen, & I. Ruoppila (Eds.). *Preparation for aging.* New York: Plenum Press, pp. 87-103.

Meerding, W., Bonneux, L., Polder, J., Koopmanschap, M.A., & Van der Maas, P.J., (1998). Demographic and epidemiological determinants of health care costs in The Netherlands: Costs of illness study. *British Medical Journal* 317, 111-115.

Netherlands Central Bureau of Statistics (NCBS) (1995). Vademecum of health statistics of the Netherlands 1995. Voorburg/Heerlen/Rijswijk: Netherlands Central Bureau of Statistics/Ministry of Health Welfare and Sports.

Pignatti, F., Castelletti, F., Metitieri, T., Zanetti, E., Marrè, A., Bianchetti, A., Rozzini, R., & Tracchi, M. (2000). Living alone and mortality in an oldest old population living at home. *The Gerontologist* 40 (Special Issue I), 365-366.

Portrait, F., Lindeboom, M., & Deeg, D. (2000a). Life expectancies in specific health states. In: F. Portrait. *Long-term care services for the Dutch Elderly. An investigation into the process of utilization.* Tinbergen Institute Research Series no. 237. Amsterdam: Thela Thesis, pp. 49-75.

Portrait, F., Lindeboom, M., & Deeg, D. (2000b). The use of long-term care services by the Dutch elderly. *Health Economics* 9, 513-531.

Radloff, L.S. (1977). The CES-D scale: A self-report depression scale for research in the general population. *Applied Psychological Measures* 1, 385-401.

Samuelsson, G., & Dehlin, O. (1993). Family network and mortality: Survival chances through the lifespan of an entire age cohort. *International Journal of Aging and Human Development* 37, 277-295.

Schellevis, F.G., Van der Velden, J., Van de Lisdonk, E., Van Eijk, J.T.M., & Van Weel, C. (1993). Comorbidity of chronic diseases in general practice. *Journal of Clinical Epidemiology* 46, 469-473.

Schiepers, J.M.P. (1988). Huishoudensequivalentiefactoren volgens de budget verdelingsmethode [Household equivalence factors using the budget distribution method]. Supplement to Sociaal-Economische Maandstatistiek 2, 28-36. In Dutch.

Smit, J.H., De Vries, M.Z. (1994). Procedures and results of the field work. In D.J.H. Deeg, & M. Westendorp-de Serière (Eds.). *Autonomy and well-being in the aging population I: Report from the Longitudinal Aging Study Amsterdam 1992-1993.* Amsterdam: VU University Press, pp. 7-13.

Smit, J.H., De Vries, M.Z., & Poppelaars, J.L. (1998). Data-collection and fieldwork procedures. In D.J.H. Deeg, A.T.F. Beekman, D.M.W. Kriegsman, & M. Westendorp- de Serière (Eds.). *Autonomy and well-being in the aging population II: Report from the Longitudinal Aging Study Amsterdam 1992-1996.* Amsterdam: VU University Press, pp. 9-20.

Tombaugh, T.N., & McIntyre, N.J. (1992). The Mini-Mental State Examination: A comprehensive review. *Journal of the American Geriatrics Society* 40, 922-935.

Valkonen, T., & Van Poppel, W.F.A. (1997). The contribution of smoking to sex differences in life expectancy: Four Nordic countries and The Netherlands. *European Journal of Public Health* 7, 302-310.

Van der Kaa, D.J. (2000). Op zoek naar Methusalem [In search of Methusalem]. Gerôn 2/3, 62-71. In Dutch.

Van Hoorn, W.D., & De Beer, J. (1997). De sterfte-hypothese in de nationale bevolking sprognose van 1996 [The mortality hypothesis in the 1996 national population prognosis]. In A. van den Berg Jeths (Ed.). Volksgezondheid Toekomst Verkenning 1997. VII. Gezondheid en zorg in de toekomst [Public Health Future

Forecast 1997. VII. Health and care in the future]. Bilthoven: National Institute for Public Health and Environment/Maarssen: Elsevier-De Tijdstroom, 81-90. In Dutch.

Van Poppel, F., & De Beer, J. (1996). Evaluation of standard mortality projections for the elderly. In G. Caselli, & A.D. Lopez (Eds.). *Health and mortality among elderly populations*. Oxford: Clarendon Press, pp. 288-315.

Van Sonsbeek, J.L.A. (1988). Methodische en inhoudelijke aspecten van de OESO-vragenlijst betreffende langdurige beperkingen in het lichamelijk functioneren [Methodological and substantial aspects of the OECD questionnaire regarding long-term limitations in physical functioning]. Maandbericht Gezondheid (CBS) 88/6, 4-17. In Dutch.

Verbrugge, L.M. (1985). Gender and health: An update on hypotheses and evidence. *Journal of Health and Social Behavior* 26, 156-182.

Verheij, R.A. (1996). Explaining urban-rural variations in health: A review of interactions between individual and environment. *Social Science and Medicine* 42, 923-935.

Verkleij, H., & Mackenbach, J.P. (1998). "Volksgezondheid toekomst verkenning," 1997. III. Gezondheidsverschillen in Nederland ["Public health future forecast," 1997. III. Health differentials in the Netherlands]. *Nederlands Tijdschrift voor Geneeskunde* 142, 1219-1223. In Dutch.

Wenger, N.K. (1998). An update on coronary heart disease in women. *International Journal of Fertility and Women's Medicine* 43, 84-90.

Wilson, R.W., & McNeil, J.M. (1981). Preliminary analysis of OECD disability on the pretest of the post census disability survey. *Revue Epidémiologie et Santé Publique* 29, 469-75.

Life With and Without Disease:
Women Experience More of Both

Eileen M. Crimmins, PhD
Jung Ki Kim, PhD
Aaron Hagedorn, BS

SUMMARY. This paper examines gender differences in life with and without six major diseases, including both mortal and morbid conditions. Disease prevalence and health behavior data are from the 1993-1995 National Health Interview Surveys for the United States. Vital registration data are the source of mortality rates used in computing life expectancy. The Sullivan method is used to estimate life lived with and without disease and risky behavior for men and women at various ages. Women live more years with each of the diseases examined, and, for arthritis, the extended years with disease are greatest. Women also live more years than men free of each of these diseases with the exception of arthritis. Gender differences in life without two health-risk behaviors are also discussed. Men spend more years of their lives overweight and have fewer years during which they see a doctor. *[Article copies available for a fee from The Haworth Document Delivery Service: 1-800-HAWORTH.*

Eileen M. Crimmins is Edna M. Jones Professor of Gerontology and Sociology at the Andrus Gerontology Center of the University of Southern California, and Director of the USC/UCLA Center on Biodemography and Population Health, Los Angeles, CA 90089-0191.

Jung Ki Kim is a post doctoral fellow at the Andrus Gerontology Center of the University of Southern California.

Aaron Hagedorn is a doctoral student in the Leonard Davis School of Gerontology of the University of Southern California.

[Haworth co-indexing entry note]: "Life With and Without Disease: Women Experience More of Both." Crimmins, Eileen M., Jung Ki Kim, and Aaron Hagedorn. Co-published simultaneously in *Journal of Women & Aging* (The Haworth Press, Inc.) Vol. 14, No. 1/2, 2002, pp. 47-59; and: *Health Expectations for Older Women: International Perspectives* (ed: Sarah B. Laditka) The Haworth Press, Inc., 2002, pp. 47-59. Single or multiple copies of this article are available for a fee from The Haworth Document Delivery Service [1-800-HAWORTH 9:00 a.m. - 5:00 p.m. (EST). E-mail address: getinfo@haworthpressinc.com].

47

E-mail address: <getinfo@haworthpressinc.com> Website: <http://www. HaworthPress.com> © 2002 by The Haworth Press, Inc. All rights reserved.]

KEYWORDS. Healthy life expectancy, chronic diseases, gender differences

INTRODUCTION

Most research on active life expectancy has focused on life with and without disability (Branch et al., 1991; Crimmins et al., 1996, 1997; Crimmins and Saito, 2001; Manton and Stallard, 1991). This paper moves further back in the process of health change to examine gender differences in life with and without major diseases and differences in years with two health risk behaviors. A number of national and international groups have recognized the value of multiple approaches to measuring healthy life expectancy based on the multiple dimensions of health (World Health Organization, 1984). One reason to focus on diseases is that these are the conditions that often underlie disability and are the ultimate causes of death (Verbrugge and Jette, 1994). An additional reason for the focus on disease is that most medical care is directed at the treatment of underlying diseases; thus, the length of time lived with diagnosed disease is one factor determining the use of medical care, particularly prescription drugs. Gender differences in the length of healthy and diseased lives have implications for differential quality of life as well as resource utilization. Gender differences in the length of life with health risks are important in pointing to potential explanations for differential health outcomes.

BACKGROUND

Men and women have different patterns of both mortality and disease experience. The mortality of men exceeds the mortality of women at every age (National Center for Health Statistics, 1996). There are also marked gender differences in the age-specific pattern of disease prevalence. Men have higher prevalences of what can be termed mortal conditions like heart disease, while women are more likely to have higher prevalences of morbid conditions like arthritis (Verbrugge, 1986, 1989, 1990). Gender differences in disease presence and mortality are explained by a combination of social, behavioral, psychological, and biological factors (Nathanson, 1984).

How these factors combine to produce healthy and diseased life expectancy is the subject of this paper. Any state of health can be used as a basis for computing healthy life expectancy–or years without some adverse health state. Estimates of life with and without disability have generally shown that women's generally longer life consists of more years without disability, as well as more with disability (Branch et al., 1991; Crimmins et al., 1996; Hayward and Heron, 1999; Manton and Stallard, 1991). Differential mortality resulting in longer lives for women rather than a higher incidence of disability among women is the reason older women spend more years with disability (Crimmins et al., 1996).

Disability is an indicator of one dimension of health, the ability to perform socially accepted roles. Disability is also an end point in a process which often begins with the onset of disease (Verbrugge and Jette, 1994). Measures of the length of life with and without disease provide an additional indicator of how gender differences in health cumulate over the life cycle. Knowledge of differential disease burden in the population is very useful for health planners because most health treatment is disease-based. Major chronic diseases increasingly are treated pharmaceutically from the time of diagnosis until the time of death. Knowing how many years of treatment are likely to be required after diagnosis and being able to estimate how this would change with change in mortality rates or treatment and prevention provide valuable tools for health planners.

DATA AND METHODS

Data on the age-specific prevalence of diseases and health conditions come from the 1993-1995 U.S. National Health Interview Surveys. This is an annual survey designed to provide information on the nation's health and health care usage. Disease prevalence is determined by dividing the sample into six parts and asking one sixth of the sample about a set of diseases representing one bodily system; thus people were not asked about multiple systems. In order to make the sample large enough for stable age-specific disease prevalence estimates, information on the prevalence of diseases is based on respondents from 1993, 1994, and 1995 surveys. In each of the years, the sample was more than 100,000 persons from almost 50,000 households. This annual sample is representative of community-dwelling persons in the United States (Adams and Marano, 1995).

The questions used to estimate disease prevalence take the forms, "Has anyone in the family ever had hypertension (heart disease)" or "During the last 12 months has anyone had asthma (bronchitis or emphysema, diabetes, arthritis)" (Adams and Marano, 1995). We examine differences in the length of life with six diseases or conditions: heart disease, diabetes, hypertension, asthma, bronchitis/emphysema, and arthritis. These diseases were chosen because they are major causes of mortality and morbidity. The age-specific disease prevalences for 5-year age groups used here were determined using individual level data for those 30 and above and published data for those less than 30. In addition to information on diseases, we also include information on height and weight and on the use of medical care which is collected in the 1994 survey. We use this information to determine the age-specific prevalence of being overweight and not using medical care in the past year. We define overweight as a body/mass index of greater than or equal to 25 (National Institutes of Health, 1998).

Years with and without diseases and these health risks are calculated by linking the age-specific prevalence of health states to life table estimates of the length of life lived in each age group for men and women. Information on age-sex mortality comes from the Vital Registration System (National Center for Health Statistics, 1996). The Sullivan method of constructing health expectancy is used along with software developed by Jagger (1999). This method is a cross-sectional approach which uses estimates of the prevalence of health problems at each age to weight life table estimates of years lived in each age interval into years lived with healthy and unhealthy life. For this analysis, life is divided into years with no disease or health risk and years with disease or health risk. The standard error of the estimates is used to determine whether there are gender differences in the length of healthy and unhealthy life.

RESULTS

The prevalence of disease. The age-specific prevalences of diseases for men and women are shown in Figures 1a, b, and c. Figure 1a shows the prevalence of diseases that are not very age-related: asthma and bronchitis and emphysema. In fact, asthma prevalence is highest at the younger ages and lowest among the oldest members of the population. This is a cohort rather than an age difference and reflects the worldwide

FIGURE 1a. Age-Specific Prevalence of Bronchitis or Emphysema and Asthma by Gender

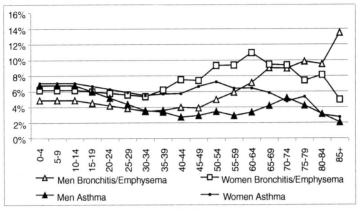

Source: 1994 National Health Interview Survey

increase in asthma in recent decades (Anderson et al., 1994). Women have slightly higher rates of asthma than men at almost all ages. Bronchitis and emphysema prevalence is fairly constant across the early part of the age range, but increases at late middle age to peak among those in their 60s. Women report more bronchitis and emphysema than men at all ages up to 75. The prevalence of bronchitis and emphysema is lower at the oldest ages for women. This is likely to reflect the increased mortality among those with these conditions.

Diabetes and hypertension (Figure 1b), heart disease and arthritis (Figure 1c) are diseases that are more age-related. Diabetes reaches prevalence levels of just over 12 percent for those in their 70s, while the other conditions reach levels of about 30 to 55 percent in old age. Diabetes and hypertension peak among those in their 70s and heart disease and arthritis among the oldest group, those in their 80s. The age-specific prevalence of diabetes is fairly similar for men and women across the age range. Women have a higher prevalence of arthritis at all ages; whereas men have a higher prevalence of heart disease at all ages over 50; on the other hand, women have a higher prevalence of hypertension after 55.

Mortality. Gender differences in age-specific survival based on the 1994 mortality rates are shown in Figure 2. The survival curve for

FIGURE 1b. Age-Specific Prevalence of Diabetes and Hypertension by Gender

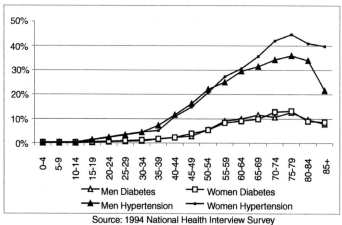

Source: 1994 National Health Interview Survey

FIGURE 1c. Age-Specific Prevalence of Arthritis and Heart Disease by Gender

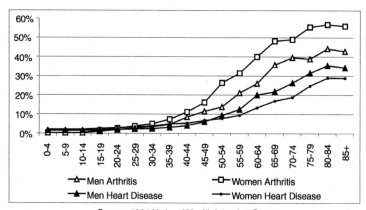

Source: 1994 National Health Interview Survey

women is above that of men indicating that a greater proportion of women in a cohort survives to each age. By age 76, only half of the original cohort of men is alive; the corresponding age for women is 82. The difference between the two survival curves reflects the longer life of women.

FIGURE 2. Probability of Survival by Gender

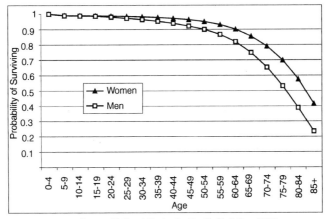

Source: National Center for Health Statistics, 1996.

Life with disease. In Table 1, information is provided on total ex-pected years of life at birth and at age 65, as well as life with and without major diseases for both men and women. The size of the gender gap along with the significance of the difference is also indicated. In 1994 in the United States, the average length of life without heart disease is 69 and the average number of years lived with heart disease is 6.7. Men live 6.3 years with heart disease while women spend 6.8 years with this condition. Looking at life without disease indicates that women have an age of heart disease onset almost 6 years later than that of men.

Arthritis is the condition that affects the total population the longest. Arthritis is a disease for which both men and women have an average age of onset of about 64; however, because women spend the rest of their longer lifespan with arthritis, the years lived with arthritis for women are almost double those of men (15.2 versus 8.8). Hypertension is the condition affecting men longer than any other condition, yet women live longer with hypertension than men. Women would require 12 years of monitoring or treatment for hypertension and men only 9.

The diseases which are not strongly associated with age–asthma and bronchitis/emphysema–have smaller gender differences in the length of diseased life. Women live just over 1.5 years longer with both of these conditions. Because diabetes prevalence is relatively low even at the

TABLE 1. Life Expectancy at Birth and Age 65, Total, Without and With Disease: 1994 United States (Standard Error in Parentheses)

	Total	Men	Women	Significance
Life Expectancy at Birth	75.7	72.6	78.8	
Without heart disease	69.0 (.10)	66.3 (.14)	72.0 (.15)	***
Without arthritis	63.5 (.12)	63.8 (.16)	63.6 (.19)	
Without diabetes	72.5 (.07)	69.9 (.10)	75.4 (.11)	***
Without hypertension	64.8 (.12)	63.4 (.16)	66.6 (.18)	***
Without asthma	71.5 (.08)	69.4 (.10)	74.0 (.12)	***
Without bronchitis/emphysema	70.7 (.09)	68.6 (.11)	73.1 (.13)	***
With heart disease	6.7 (.10)	6.3 (.14)	6.8 (.15)	*
With arthritis	12.2 (.12)	8.8 (.16)	15.2 (.19)	***
With diabetes	3.2 (.07)	2.7 (.10)	3.4 (.11)	***
With hypertension	10.9 (.12)	9.2 (.16)	12.2 (.18)	***
With asthma	4.2 (.08)	3.2 (.10)	4.8 (.12)	***
With bronchitis/emphysema	5.0 (.09)	4.0 (.11)	5.7 (.13)	***
Life Expectancy at Age 65	17.4	15.8	18.8	
Without heart disease	13.1 (.10)	11.4 (.14)	14.5 (.13)	***
Without arthritis	9.3 (.10)	9.6 (.16)	8.9 (.16)	**
Without diabetes	15.5 (.07)	14.1 (.10)	16.7 (.10)	***
Without hypertension	11.0 (.10)	10.7 (.15)	11.2 (.16)	
Without asthma	16.7 (.04)	15.2 (.06)	17.9 (.06)	***
Without bronchitis/emphysema	15.9 (.06)	14.3 (.10)	17.3 (.08)	***
With heart disease	4.3 (.10)	4.4 (.14)	4.2 (.13)	
With arthritis	8.1 (.10)	6.2 (.16)	9.9 (.16)	***
With diabetes	1.9 (.07)	1.7 (.10)	2.1 (.10)	**
With hypertension	6.4 (.10)	5.1 (.15)	7.6 (.16)	***
With asthma	0.7 (.04)	0.6 (.06)	0.9 (.06)	**
With bronchitis/emphysema	1.5 (.06)	1.5 (.10)	1.5 (.08)	

* $p < .1$ ** $p < .05$ *** $p < .001$

older ages and fairly similar for men and women, the years spent with diabetes over the life cycle only differ by 0.7 for men and women. Women still live more years on average with diabetes.

At age 65 there is no gender difference in the length of life with either heart disease or bronchitis and emphysema. Women live longer with each of the other diseases in old age. Women live longer after age 65 without each of these conditions except arthritis.

Life with health risks. Lifetime differences in health risk for men and women can also be expressed in terms of years lived with and without risky behavior. Expected years with and without a doctor visit along with years overweight, and not overweight are shown for men and women in the U.S. population in 1994 (Table 2). Both lack of medical care and obesity are risk factors for poor health outcomes including both disease onset, disability, and death. Until age 75, men are less likely to see a doctor than women (Kramarow et al., 1999). Summary indicators show that even though men live an average about 6 years less than women, they average 20 years during their lives with no doctor visit, while for women only 14 years are without a doctor visit. If an annual doctor visit is a health goal, this measure clearly indicates the gap between the current state and the goal for men. After age 65 the gender

TABLE 2. Life Expectancy With and Without at Least One Doctor Visit per Year; Expected Life Obese and Not Obese: At Birth, Ages 20 and 65 (Standard Error in Parentheses)

	Total	Men	Women	Significance
Total Expected Life at Birth	75.7	72.6	78.8	
With a Doctor Visit	58.8 (.08)	52.4 (.12)	65.2 (.10)	**
Without a Doctor Visit	16.9 (.08)	20.2 (.12)	13.6 (.10)	**
Total Expected Life at Age 20	56.9	53.9	59.7	
With BMI ≥ 25	29.1 (.10)	32.2 (.14)	25.8 (.14)	**
With BMI < 25	27.8 (.10)	21.7 (.14)	33.9 (.14)	**
Total Expected Life at Age 65	17.4	15.8	18.8	
With a Doctor Visit	15.3 (.05)	13.6 (.07)	16.7 (.07)	*
Without a Doctor Visit	2.1 (.05)	2.2 (.07)	2.1 (.07)	
With BMI ≥ 25	8.7 (.07)	8.6 (.10)	8.8 (.10)	
With BMI < 25	8.7 (.07)	7.2 (.10)	10.0 (.10)	**

*p < .05, **p < .001

difference changes: the number of years men and women do not see a doctor is similar but for women the years with a doctor visit are greater. Both men and women see a doctor during most of the years lived after age 65. Because women live longer than men, their number of years with a doctor visit is greater.

Men spend a greater number of years and proportion of their lives overweight than women. On average American men spend 32 years or 60 percent of their lives after age 20 with a body/mass index higher than 25. On average women spend fewer years, 26 years, and a smaller percentage, 43 percent, of their adult lives overweight. The number of years men and women spent being overweight is the same after age 65. Both women and men spend about 9 years after age 65, in the overweight state.

DISCUSSION

Gender differences in the length of life with disease exist for all conditions examined. Women spend more years on average with each of these diseases. Because men have a higher prevalence of heart disease in middle and the young old ages and higher mortality rates, cardiovascular disease has been thought to be a men's problem. When a life expectancy approach is used, however, women live more years on average with heart disease than men do. This makes heart disease a major problem for women as well as men. Of course, the problem for men is that they do not live long enough with their heart disease but rather they die from it. If women experienced the higher mortality rates of men, they would only spend 5.6 years with heart disease which would be less than the time spent by men. This is one indication of how the longer lives lived by women are the reason they live more years with some diseases.

This is also true for diabetes. If men and women had the same level of mortality, that of men in 1994, they would live 2.7 and 2.8 years with diabetes. It is women's additional life span that adds 0.7 years to their average length of life with diabetes.

While heart disease is thought to be a problem for men, arthritis is thought to be a woman's problem. Indeed, for women, the expected length of life with arthritis is more than twice as long as life spent with heart disease. However, even for men, the length of life with arthritis is longer than with heart disease. Hypertension is the only condition men live with longer than arthritis. The life cycle approach provided by health expectancy measures provides a different perspective on the relative importance of disease from that derived from gender differences in prevalence or incidence rates.

For both genders, the lifetime importance of asthma and bronchitis and emphysema is shown by the health expectancy figures. While these diseases are less common than the others in the population at older ages, they are higher at younger ages. Because most people with these conditions acquire them in younger life, the lifetime accumulation in years represented by the life cycle approach indicates their importance as a population health problem.

The health expectancy approach is also useful in demonstrating the cumulative lifetime pattern of poor health behaviors. Both men and women spend too many years overweight and without medical care in the United States. However, the years with health risks for men exceed those for women. Men and women might need to be targeted separately in campaigns to improve their adherence to recommended behaviors for self care and prevention.

The life expectancy approach gives some idea of the likely cumulative effect of these health risks for projected individual lifespans. Other columns of the lifetable provide information which may be more relevant from a population or public health perspective. Table 3 shows the years lived with three diseases after ages 65 and 85 for cohorts of 100,000 men and women at birth. The difference between years lived and the life expectancy measure is that life expectancy is years per person while the years lived reflects the number of persons as well as how long each lives. Because more women survive to older ages, the gender differences in years lived with disease are even greater than those in life expectancy. A cohort of women will experience 70 percent more years of life after age 65 with hypertension than a similarly sized birth cohort

TABLE 3. Number of Years Lived with Disease After Age 65 and After Age 85 by Birth Cohorts of 100,000 Men and Women

	65+		85+	
	Men	Women	Men	Women
Hypertension	380,500	649,200	30,100	98,900
Heart Disease	332,100	362,900	47,900	71,500
Arthritis	464,800	842,200	59,900	139,000

of men. After age 85, the cohort of women lives more than three times as many years with hypertension. While the gender differences in heart disease are somewhat smaller than in hypertension, more years will be spent with heart disease among a group of older women than older men. This means that the modal patient undergoing treatment for cardiovascular conditions is likely to be a woman. The population importance of arthritis is evidenced by the fact that a cohort of 100,000 women will spend almost a million years with arthritis after age 65. For a similarly sized cohort of men, half a million arthritic years will be lived. These numbers indicate the reason behind the growing demands for medical care for conditions that are highly age-related.

Disease-specific life expectancy does not have direct policy implications without considering both the adverse consequences of disease presence and the potential for eliminating either the disease or its consequences. Most of the people diagnosed with the diseases listed here would be recommended for treatment or monitoring. For instance, treatment to reduce pain and improve mobility is usually recommended for arthritis. This treatment is relatively inexpensive and should lead to reductions in associated disability. Clearly, improvements in arthritis treatment or prevention will benefit women more than men.

Once a person has been diagnosed with hypertension, drug treatment is commonly prescribed. In fact, recently, there has been discussion of lowering the blood pressure level at which drug treatment is recommended for older people. After age 65, women spend about 50 percent more time with hypertension than men. This means that expenditures for drugs to treat this condition are likely to be more for women. Coverage of drugs under Medicare would thus improve the ability of women to cope with this condition more than men.

REFERENCES

Adams, P.F. and Marano, M.A. (1995). *Vital and Health Statistics: Current estimates from the National Health Interview Survey, 1994.* Hyattsville, MD. 10 (193). DHHS publication number (PHS) 96-1521.

Anderson, H.R., Butland, B.K., and Strachan, D.P. (1994). Trends in prevalence and severity of childhood asthma. *British Medical Journal* 308, 1600-1604.

Branch, L.G., Guralnik, J.M., Foley, D.J., Kohout, F.J., and Wetle, A.O. (1991). Active life expectancy for 10,000 Caucasian men and women in three communities. *Journal of Gerontology* 46 (4), M145-150.

Crimmins, E.M., Hayward, M.D., and Saito, Y. (1996). Differentials in active life expectancy in the older population of the United States. *Journal of Gerontology*, 51B (3), S111-120.

Crimmins, E.M. and Saito, Y. (2001). Trends in healthy life expectancy in the United States, 1970-1990: Gender, racial, and educational differences. *Social Science and Medicine* 52 (11), 1629-1641.

Crimmins, E.M., Saito, Y., and Ingegneri, D. (1997). Trends in disability-free life expectancy in the United States, 1970-90. *Population and Development Review* 23 (3), 555-572.

Hayward, M.D. and Heron, M. (1999). Racial inequality in active life expectancy among adult Americans. *Demography* 36 (1), 77-91.

Jagger, C. (1999). Health expectancy calculation by the Sullivan Method: A practical guide. European Concerted Action on the Harmonization of Health Expectancy Calculations in Europe (EURO-REVES). Nihon University Population Research Institute Research Paper Series No. 68. Tokyo, Japan.

Kramarow, E., Lentzner, H., Rooks, R., Weeks, J., and Sayah, S. (1999). *Health and Aging Chartbook. Health, United States, 1999.* Hyattsville, MD: National Center for Health Statistics, PHS 99-1232.

Manton, K.G. and Stallard, E. (1991). Cross-sectional estimates of active life expectancy for the U.S. elderly and oldest-old populations. *Journal of Gerontology* 46 (3), S170-182.

Nathanson, C.A. (1984). Sex differentials in mortality. *Annual Review of Sociology* 10, 191-213.

National Center for Health Statistics. (1996, March 19). Deaths from each cause by 5-year age groups, race and sex: United States 1994. [Online]. Available: *http://www.cdc.gov/nchs/data/gmwk1_94.pdf* [page 111]

National Institutes of Health. (1998). Clinical guideline on the identification, evaluation and treatment of overweight and obesity in adults–The evidence report. *Obesity Research* 6 (Suppl. 2), 51S-209S.

Verbrugge, L.M. (1990). Pathways of health and death. *Women, Health and Medicine in America, A Historical Handbook.* R.D. Apple. Garland, New York, 41-79.

Verbrugge, L.M. (1989). The twain meet: Empirical explanations of sex differences in health and mortality. *Journal of Health and Social Behavior* 30 (3), 282-304.

Verbrugge, L.M. (1986). From sneezes to adieux: Stages of health for American men and women. *Social Science and Medicine* 22 (11), 1195-1212.

Verbrugge, L.M. and Jette, A.M. (1994). The disablement process. *Social Science and Medicine* 38 (1), 1-14.

World Health Organization. (1984). The uses of epidemiology in the study of the elderly. *Report of a Scientific Group on the Epidemiology of Aging.* Technical Report Series, 706. Geneva: WHO.

Gender Differences in Disability-Free Life Expectancy for Selected Risk Factors and Chronic Conditions in Canada

Alain Bélanger, PhD
Laurent Martel, MSc
Jean-Marie Berthelot, BSc
Russell Wilkins, MUrb

SUMMARY. This article shows how mortality and morbidity patterns differ for women and men 45 years of age and older. The impact on disability-free life expectancy was calculated for selected risk factors and chronic conditions: low income, low education, abnormal body mass index, lack of physical activity, smoking, cancer, diabetes, and arthritis. For each factor, the expected number of years free of disability was calculated for men and women using multi-state life tables. In terms of disability-free life expectancy, the greatest impacts on affected women were for diabetes (14.1 years), arthritis (8.8 years), and physical inactivity (6.0 years), while for affected men, the greatest impacts were for dia-

Alain Bélanger and Laurent Martel are affiliated with the Demography Division, while Jean-Marie Berthelot and Russell Wilkins are with the Health Analysis and Modeling Group, Statistics Canada, Ottawa, ON, Canada, K1A 0T6.

Address correspondence to: Alain Bélanger, Demography Division, Statistics Canada, Ottawa, ON, Canada K1A 0T6 (E-mail: alain.belanger@statcan.ca).

The views and opinions expressed in this paper do not necessarily reflect those of Statistics Canada.

The authors are grateful to Health Canada for funding, and to Kathy White for editorial assistance.

[Haworth co-indexing entry note]: "Gender Differences in Disability-Free Life Expectancy for Selected Risk Factors and Chronic Conditions in Canada." Bélanger et al. Co-published simultaneously in *Journal of Women & Aging* (The Haworth Press, Inc.) Vol. 14, No. 1/2, 2002, pp. 61-83; and: *Health Expectations for Older Women: International Perspectives* (ed: Sarah B. Laditka) The Haworth Press, Inc., 2002, pp. 61-83. Single or multiple copies of this article are available for a fee from The Haworth Document Delivery Service [1-800-HAWORTH 9:00 a.m. - 5:00 p.m. (EST). E-mail address: getinfo@haworthpressinc.com].

betes (10.5 years), smoking (6.9 years), arthritis (6.5 years), and cancer (6.4 years). The implications of these results are discussed from the perspective of developing programs designed to improve population health status. *[Article copies available for a fee from The Haworth Document Delivery Service: 1-800-HAWORTH. E-mail address: <getinfo@haworthpressinc.com> Website: <http://www.HaworthPress.com> © 2002 by The Haworth Press, Inc. All rights reserved.]*

KEYWORDS. Mortality, morbidity, disability-free life expectancy, risk factors, gender differences

INTRODUCTION

In Canada, as in many other developed nations, gender differences in health present somewhat of a paradox. On the one hand, life expectancy for Canadian women has been greater than for Canadian men for over a century–81.4 and 75.8 years, respectively, in 1997 (Statistics Canada, 2001a). On the other, Canadian women reported more chronic conditions, and they used health care services more frequently, particularly at ages 65 and over (Statistics Canada, 2001b). They also had higher rates of disability (Statistics Canada, 2000). Thus, while women certainly live longer than men, their health is not as good.

Life expectancy is often used alone as an aggregate indicator for describing the health of a population or its component groups, based on the assumption that expansion of life expectancy implies better health.[1] It is tempting to consider the health of men, with a life expectancy 5.6 years less than that of women, to be the greater concern and thus the focus of more attention by public decision makers involved in defining health policies. Mortality and morbidity are, however, two distinct measures that may, in fact, provide quite opposite perspectives.

In an aging society in which the majority of seniors are women, who report more disabling chronic conditions (Manton, 1997), we need other aggregate indicators of health that provide information on both mortality and morbidity. One such indicator, disability-free life expectancy, can be used to qualify years of life according to whether they are with or without disability. In so doing, this aggregate health indicator sheds more meaning on longer life by helping to determine whether an increase in average lifespan is accompanied by better quality of life. Once this indicator has been estimated for both sexes, it can demonstrate how the aging of men and women differs in terms of functional health. In the short term, as accelerated aging of the Canadian population threatens to trigger a significant rise in costs for health care and related services, living not just longer, but in better health and while maintaining physical autonomy, would appear to be a desirable goal. Strategies aimed at compression of morbidity, which may be different for each sex, thus warrant special attention.

This research assesses the effects of various risk factors and chronic conditions on disability-free life expectancy for Canadian men and women. In a prior study, numerous factors were significantly associated with the loss and recovery of functional autonomy (Martel, Bélanger, and Berthelot, 2000). The current study compares the effect of several of these factors (education and income as social factors; physical activity, body mass index, and smoking as behavioural factors; arthritis, diabetes, and cancer as chronic conditions) on the life expectancy and disability-free life expectancy of Canadian men and women. To our knowledge, there has been no other study on this subject for Canada.

Because functional health is a dynamic process, i.e., a person who has lost physical autonomy could subsequently recover it, the method used here to calculate disability-free life expectancy is based on multi-state life tables. More complex than the well-known "Sullivan" prevalence-based method, this method considers the flow into and out of disability, referred to as "transitions between functional states." This method also allows for explicit differences in mortality between different functional health states. A longitudinal survey is necessary to calculate these transitions and in this case the Canadian National Population Health Survey (NPHS) was used. The NPHS is the first longitudinal survey designed to enhance understanding of the processes affecting the health of the Canadian population as a whole, including persons living in private households and health-related institutions.

BACKGROUND

To our knowledge, few studies have estimated the impact of various health risk factors and chronic conditions on disability-free life expectancy, particularly by using the multi-state method. Various work has, however, been conducted to examine the effect on disability-free life expectancy of smoking (Rogers et al., 1994; Nusselder, 1998; Ferrucci et al., 1999), physical activity (Ferrucci et al., 1999), certain chronic illnesses (Nusselder, 1998), marital status (Nault et al., 1996), and socioeconomic status (Guralnik et al., 1993; Leigh and Fries, 1994; Wigle, 1995; Nault et al., 1996; Valkonen et al., 1997; Doblhammer and Kytir, 1998; Melzer et al., 2000).

Many studies have highlighted the links between socio-economic status and health. The higher the educational or income level, the greater life expectancy and better health. Melzer et al. (2000) showed that a higher educational level was associated with a relative compression of morbidity, as members of higher social classes not only enjoyed longer life expectancies, but also a greater proportion of such years lived in good health. Similar results were also reported by Leigh and Fries (1994) and Doblhammer and Kytir (1998). Valkonen et al. (1997), however, reported that the number of years lived with disability remained higher among women than among men whatever the educational level, both because of their longer life expectancies and their likelihood of disability.

According to Nault et al. (1996), differences between Canadian men and women with respect to mortality and morbidity diminished with increasing socioeconomic status. In another study of the Canadian population, Wigle (1995) showed that disability-free life expectancy in Canada was much lower for individuals falling into the bottom income quintile compared with those in the top (a difference of 10.1 years for men and 11.3 years for women). Differences in mortality and morbidity by socioeconomic status thus persist in Canada, despite the principles of universal coverage and accessibility that underpin Canada's health care system.

With respect to behaviours affecting mortality and health, all studies on smoking have demonstrated the extent to which it contributes to mortality and morbidity. Ferrucci et al. (1999), Nusselder (1998), and Bronnum-Hansen and Juel (2001) showed clearly that a lower prevalence of smoking resulted not only in longer life expectancy and disability-free life expectancy, but also reduced the proportion of life lived with disability. In other words, smoking reduction led to a relative compression of morbidity. Ferrucci et al. (1999) showed that regular physical activity also yielded the same result.

Few studies have assessed the impact of chronic illnesses on both mortality and morbidity. Using an approach different than the one employed in our research, Mathers (1992) and Nusselder (1998) illustrated the effect of eliminating a given illness on life expectancy and on disability-free life expectancy.[2] She concluded that eliminating non-fatal chronic illnesses, such as arthritis and back pain, would lead to a substantial rise in disability-free life expectancy, without significantly increasing life expectancy. This means that efforts to eliminate these diseases could produce an absolute compression of morbidity. On the other hand, the elimination of more fatal diseases like cancer or heart disease could lead to an expansion of morbidity, as their impact on life expectancy alone was much greater than on disability-free life expectancy.

More recently, Laditka and Laditka (2001) have shown that iniviuals suffering from diabetes can expect to live fewer years of both total and unimpaired life, indicating that this chronic disease has a major impact on health expectancy.

The calculation of indicators such as disability-free life expectancy or healthy life expectancy requires access to detailed health surveys and is not yet very widespread, particularly using the multi-state life table method. Simultaneously comparing the impact of multiple risk factors and chronic conditions on disability-free life expectancy computed through this method is thus a first in largely uncharted territory. This means we will not be able to directly compare our results here with those presented in our survey of the literature.

DATA AND METHODS

The National Population Health Survey (NPHS) was launched by Statistics Canada in 1994. It provides both cross-sectional and longitudinal data on the population living in private households and those living in health-related institutions. Its longitudinal dimension involves interviewing respondents every two years to gather detailed information on their physical and mental health, activity limitations and disabilities, use of and access to health care, chronic health problems, lifestyle, and health-related behaviours.

The NPHS longitudinal sample included 17,276 respondents living in private households and 2,192 living in health-related institutions in 1994. As our study was restricted to individuals 45 years of age or older,[3] 6,053 respondents in private households and 1,956 in institutions were selected from the initial sample. Only the first two NPHS cycles (1994 and 1996) were used. Loss to follow-up between 1994 and 1996 was very low, and did not constitute a major source of bias.[4]

Functional Health States

Health as a concept is difficult to define because it involves more than just the absence of disease. By defining health as a functional state that either does or does not permit autonomy in activities of daily living, we can then link health status to its potential burden on the formal and/or informal support network.

Operationally, two concepts were used and combined under the generic term "disability" in order to define an individual's functional state: activity limitations and dependency. In the first state, respondents were considered to be "disability-free" if they reported no activity limitations and no dependency. The second state of "slight or moderate disability" included respondents who had some activity limitations but no dependency, or who needed assistance from someone for heavy household chores, shopping or normal everyday housework, whether or not they reported any activity limitations. Individuals with "severe disabilities" are those who required assistance from another person in preparing their meals, in providing their personal care, or in helping them get about the house, whether or not they also had any activity limitations. Finally, residents of long-term health-related facilities constituted the fourth functional state: "institutionalization."

A higher proportion of women than men 45 years or older were classified as disabled (Table 1), suggesting poorer functional health among the female population. Women reported more disabling chronic diseases than men and were also older on average (Statistics Canada, 2000). Relatively few men reported that they needed outside help in preparing their meals, shopping, or for normal everyday housework, suggesting that dependency in these tasks may be related to the

TABLE 1. Definitions of the Four Functional States and Their Prevalence in the Canadian Population Aged 45 and Over, by Sex, 1995

Functional State	Activity Limitations	Dependency	Prevalence (%)		
			Men	Women	Total
Disability-free	None	None	72.8	66.9	69.7
Slight or moderate disability	Yes	No			
	Yes or no	Heavy household chores, shopping for groceries, normal everyday housework	20.8	24.5	22.7
Severe disability	Yes or no	Meals preparation, personal care, moving around the house	5.1	5.9	5.5
Institutionalization	--	Residence in a long-term health-related facility	1.3	2.8	2.0

gender division of household work, at least for the generations under study. The use of "activity limitations," which is less sensitive to traditional gender roles, allowed us to reduce its impact on observed prevalence, thus making it easier to create relatively homogeneous functional states that included enough cases to yield reliable estimates.

Risk Factors

Table 2 defines the risk factors and chronic conditions examined and their prevalence within the study population. Respondents' education was categorized as "high school graduation or less" or as "at least some post-secondary." The proportion of women with a lower educational level was only slightly higher than that of men, which was to be expected among the generations under study.

The income variable divided the population into two groups with cut-offs which varied according to the number of people living in the household: "low income" and "middle or high income" were defined as in Table 2. Almost one in four women lived in a low income household, while this was only true of about one in seven men. Once again, these results have been affected by the generational factor, as many older women did not join the workforce during what would have been their working lives. Given the relationship between health and socioeconomic status, women, who tended to have less education and lower income than men, were at a disadvantage when it comes to risk factors for health.

In this study, a respondent who reported being a daily smoker, an occasional but formerly daily smoker or a former smoker who had stopped within the prior five years, was classified as a smoker, since there is a latency period for many smoking-related diseases. Conversely, respondents who had never smoked, who had stopped smoking more than five years earlier or who were always only occasional smokers were classified as non-smokers. About one in three men aged 45 or older fell into the smoker category. Among women the proportion was only one in four. Note also that relatively few women now in the older age groups smoked before the 1970s.

Body mass index (BMI) was obtained by dividing an individual's weight in kilograms by the square of his or her height in metres. Various standards define underweight and obesity, the most common being the World Health Organization definition of underweight as a BMI of $\leq$ 18.5 and obese as $\geq$ 30.0 (WHO, 1995). We chose a different approach here, which began by classifying the population into deciles of BMI by

TABLE 2. Definitions of the Various Risk Factors and Chronic Conditions and Their Prevalence in the Canadian Population Aged 45 and Over, by Sex, 1995

Risk factor or chronic condition	Definition	Prevalence (%)		
		Men	Women	Total
Education				
Lower education	High school graduation or less	51.3	55.3	53.4
Higher education	At least some post-secondary education	48.7	44.7	46.6
Income*				
Low income	Less than $15,000 for a one or two person household Less than $20,000 for a three or four person household Less than $30,000 for a five or more person household	14.4	23.6	19.3
Middle or high income	At least $15,000 for a one or two person household At least $20,000 for a three or four person household At least $30,000 for a five or more person household	85.6	76.4	80.7
Smoking				
Smoker	Daily smoker Occasional smoker but former daily smoker Former smoker who stopped less than 5 years ago	31.8	23.9	27.6
Non-smoker	Always an occasional smoker Former smoker who stopped more than 5 years ago Never a smoker	68.2	76.1	72.4
Body Mass Index				
Abnormal BMI	Deciles 1 and 10 for age group and sex	20.0	20.0	20.0
Normal BMI	Deciles 2 to 9 for age group and sex	80.0	80.0	80.0
Physical Activity**				
Inactive	Less than 1.5 kcal/kg/day of energy expenditure	61.9	67.2	64.8
Active	1.5 kcal/kg/day or more of energy expenditure	38.1	32.8	35.2
Arthritis				
Yes	Arthritis ever diagnosed by a health professional	21.1	33.3	27.7
No	Never diagnosed with arthritis	78.9	66.7	72.3
Diabetes				
Yes	Diabetes ever diagnosed by a health professional	7.3	6.2	6.7
No	Never diagnosed with diabetes	92.7	93.8	93.3
Cancer				
Yes	Cancer ever diagnosed by a health professional	2.8	4.3	3.6
No	Never diagnosed with cancer	97.2	95.7	96.4

*Household income for persons living in private households; personal income for persons residing in health-related institutions.
**Leisure time physical activity.

age and sex. Individuals falling into the extreme lower or upper deciles (the first or tenth) were considered to be of "abnormal" weight.[5] This method resulted in no difference in prevalence by sex, since by definition, 20% of both men and women would be of abnormal weight.

The NPHS was used to calculate total cumulative energy expenditure of respondents during their leisure activities based on their weight and duration of leisure activities during the three months preceding the interview. Active individuals were those who expended more than 1.5 kilocalories per kilogram of body mass per day, which corresponds to moderate or intense physical activity. In our sample, somewhat more men than women were physically active according to this definition, which also corresponds to results generally appearing in reports on men's and women's health (Statistics Canada, 2000).

Finally, concerning chronic conditions, respondents were asked if a health care professional had ever diagnosed them with one of a list of various health-related problems.[6] Based on these questions, the respondent was categorized as ever or never diagnosed with arthritis, diabetes, or cancer. The survey questionnaire did not provide any additional information on the type or severity of the disease (such as whether diabetes was type I or type II).

The prevalence of diabetes and cancer was similar among both sexes in the population aged 45 and older. Arthritis, however, presented fairly different profiles for each sex, with far more women (one in three) than men (one in five) reporting that they had been diagnosed with this chronic condition.

Methods

The calculation of disability-free life expectancy using multi-state life tables is based on estimating two elements: the first is the mortality differential by functional state and risk factor or chronic condition and the second is the transitions between the different functional states for the populations with and without the risk factor or chronic condition.

Since the NPHS sample was relatively small, estimating mortality rates by age, sex, and the four functional states did not produce very robust results using only the survey data. However, life tables produced from the vital statistics provided a better estimate of mortality for the Canadian population as a whole. The method used to estimate the mortality differential by functional state took advantage of this information and used the survey data to increase or decrease the risk of death of individuals according to their functional state reported in the first cycle by means of an estimation of relative risks. Obtained by using a proportional hazard model (Cox regression),[7] these relative risks for each of the states were applied to the probability of dying from the Canadian life tables (based on vital statistics) to produce new probabilities of dying for each functional state. The mortality base level was, therefore, a reliable estimate that took the whole of the Canadian population into consideration. For each risk factor or chronic condition, the respective prevalences were used in combination with these new probabilities of dying to generate a new life table for the total population which showed approximately the same life expectancy obtained using the reference Canadian life tables based on vital statistics.

Because of the small sample size, the direct calculation of the probability of making a transition between each functional state–by age, sex, and risk factor or chronic condition–would introduce undesirable random variations from one age group to another. Instead, transitions between functional states by age and sex for each risk factor and chronic condition were estimated using a generalized logit model[8] which eliminated those random variations. For each original functional state, the probability of making a transition to another state was assumed to be a function of age and sex, the only two variables included in the regression. The model provided for inclusion of competing risks, that is, that the probability of making a transition from one functional state to another also depended on all of the other states. These transitions were modelled for each of the various risk factors and chronic condition categories. We assumed that individuals who died between 1994 and 1996 lived half that time (one year). Results are presented for 1995, halfway through the interval between the first two NPHS cycles.

To simplify the reporting of results, "disabled life expectancy" (DLE or DLE *Any* in the tables) includes moderate disability, severe disability, and institutionalization, while "severely disabled life expectancy" (DLE *Severe* in the tables) includes severe disability and institutionalization.

RESULTS

Table 3 presents life expectancy and disability-free life expectancy in years, by sex, for each risk factor and chronic condition studied. The years lived with severe disability or in a health-related institution are also provided. Total life expectancy at age 45, as estimated by the multi-state life table method, was 32.9 years for men and 37.7 years for women in 1995 (Table 3). By comparison, life expectancy at the same age according to the official Statistics Canada life tables based on vital statistics was 32.7 years for men and 37.6 years for women (Bélanger, 1999). The estimate of life expectancy based on the method used here thus seems to be fairly accurate, given the random variation due to use of data from a sample-based survey.

TABLE 3. Life Expectancy (LE), Disability-Free Life Expectancy (DFLE), and Disabled Life Expectancy (DLE) at Age 45 for the Total Population and for Selected Risk Factors and Chronic Conditions, by Sex, Canada, 1995 (Multi-State Model)

	Men				Women			
	LE	DFLE	DLE		LE	DFLE	DLE	
Risk factor or chronic condition			*Any*	*Severe*			*Any*	*Severe*
Total population	32.9	22.3	10.6	2.3	37.7	22.6	15.1	3.7
Education								
Lower education	30.9	20.8	10.1	2.3	36.2	21.5	14.3	3.7
Higher education	37.2	25.2	12.0	2.0	42.3	24.7	17.8	3.6
Income								
Low income	30.3	20.2	10.1	3.3	33.7	19.2	14.5	4.1
Middle or high income	33.6	22.8	10.8	2.0	37.5	23.7	3.8	2.2
Smoking								
Smoker	28.1	17.8	10.3	2.3	30.4	17.0	13.4	3.2
Non-smoker	35.5	24.7	10.7	2.3	40.8	25.0	15.8	3.9
Body Mass Index (BMI)								
Abnormal BMI	30.2	22.8	7.4	2.3	32.1	20.3	11.8	3.5
Normal BMI	33.8	22.5	11.3	2.3	39.6	23.6	15.8	3.8
Physical activity								
Inactive	31.9	22.0	9.9	2.0	36.7	21.6	15.1	3.5
Active	35.8	24.4	11.4	1.8	43.6	27.6	16.0	2.8
Arthritis								
Yes	31.1	16.7	14.3	2.8	35.4	15.8	19.6	4.2
No	33.3	23.2	10.1	2.4	38.7	24.6	14.1	4.0
Diabetes								
Yes	27.7	12.0	15.7	12.3	26.0	9.2	16.8	4.7
No	33.3	22.7	10.6	2.3	39.0	23.3	15.7	3.8
Cancer								
Yes	23.0	16.4	6.6	1.5	26.1	17.8	8.3	2.8
No	34.0	22.8	11.2	2.5	39.0	23.1	15.9	4.1

Note. DLE *Any* includes any disability or institutionalization; DLE *Severe* includes severe disability or institutionalization

Of the two socio-economic factors appearing in Table 3, differences between low and high educational levels produced the larger effects with respect to mortality: nearly 6 years of life expectancy for both men and women. By contrast, differences between the lower and higher income levels were 3.3 years for men and 3.8 years for women. The more marked effect of educational level can be explained largely by the fact that life expectancies of well-educated individuals were particularly high. In addition to the link with prevalences indicated in Table 2, this probably reflected strong relationships between educational level and health-related behaviours (Millar and Stephens, 1992). Furthermore, the Canadian health system is based on principles of universality and accessibility, probably limiting the impact of low income on health.

With respect to morbidity, nearly all additional years of life expectancy for those with higher income were disability-free years. Consequently, there was little difference in the number of years lived with disability across the two income categories, although life expectancy was much shorter for persons with low income. By income, expected years of life with disability were 10.8 years versus 10.1 years among men and 14.5 years versus 13.8 among women. Low-income individuals, however, spent more time with severe disabilities or in health-related institutions–an additional 1.3 years for men and 1.9 years for women–despite their shorter life expectancy.

By sex, income-related loss of disability-free years was greater among low-income women than among low-income men (4.5 years less for women versus 2.6 years less for men) although the reverse was found with respect to educational levels (3.2 years less for women versus 4.4 years less for men). This phenomenon is probably due to the greater attention women pay to their health and their greater exposure to precarious financial situations. The latter factor would discriminate more with respect to the income variable than to the educational level.

Smoking had a dramatic effect on both mortality and morbidity. Cancer, for both sexes, and diabetes among women had greater impacts on life expectancy. Among men, the difference in life expectancy between smokers and non-smokers was more than 7 years. This difference climbed to over 10 years among women (Table 3)–over one quarter of their remaining life expectancy. This greater impact of smoking on women was also reported by Prescott et al. (1999) and was attributed to the differential trends in smoking prevalence by sex within the generations under study. Men began smoking in large numbers earlier than women and many stopped during the course of their lives. As a result, the population of non-smoking men had a larger proportion of former smokers compared with women, among whom the widespread use of tobacco began much later.[9]

The impact of smoking was not limited to mortality: almost all (95%) of the additional years a male non-smoker could expect to live, compared with a smoker, were likely to be lived free of disability. Not only did smokers thus risk dying younger than non-smokers, but on average they also risked becoming limited in their daily activities earlier than did non-smokers. For individual women, the gains in disability-free life expectancy related to not smoking were slightly greater than those of men, but they represented a smaller proportion (77%) of gains in life expectancy. As life expectancies of non-smokers were much higher than those of smokers, non-smokers could expect slightly more years with disability than smokers. A similar pattern was reported above for educational level.

The impact on mortality of two other behavioural factors, physical activity and body mass index, was similar. For each, there was a difference in life expectancy of 4 years among men and of about 7 years among women. The link between physical inactivity and excess weight or obesity is well known (Chen and Millar, 2001): individuals with excess weight or obesity are less likely to be active or to start exercising. One would expect that underweight individuals, and particularly women, have higher mortality levels, especially after age 65, when weight loss and disease often go hand in hand. Furthermore, the predominantly female population living in health-related institutions was assumed to be inactive; the combined effect with the greater inactivity of women in the private household population helps to explain why women are more prone to mortality associated with these two behavioural factors.

Compared with normal body mass index, abnormal body mass index had no impact on disability-free life expectancy among men (again of 0.3 years) but a large impact among women (a loss of 3.3 years). However, among both sexes, differences were much greater for physical inactivity (a loss of 2.4 years among men and 6.0 years among women). About 60% of the additional life expectancy for physically active men was disability-free. These figures rose to 85% among women.

Of the three chronic conditions examined, arthritis had by far the smallest impact on the mortality of both men and women: losses in life expectancy were 2.2 years for men and 3.3 years for women. However, the impact was much greater on morbidity. For individuals with arthritis, disability-free life expectancy was reduced by nearly 9 years among women and more than 6 years among men. Women with arthritis on average spent more of their remaining years with disability than without (19.6 years with disability versus 15.8 years without disability), a pattern that was not observed among men who had arthritis or any other risk factor or chronic condition. Eliminating arthritis would thus result in both an absolute and relative compression of morbidity as there would be fewer years with disability while life expectancy would also increase slightly.

Diabetes had a strong impact on both mortality and morbidity. Of the risk factors and chronic conditions presented here, diabetes appeared to be the most damaging to health. It took more years of life among women than did cancer or smoking, the two other factors with very strong impacts on mortality. The effect of diabetes on male mortality was less marked than that of cancer, smoking, or low education. Similar differences in loss of life expectancy between the sexes were also found by Geiss et al. (2001), and probably have their origins in links between diabetes and heart disease (Giardina, 2000), a link considered to take a heavier toll among women (Keller and Lemberg, 2000). The lesser effect of cancer among women may be due to the high prevalence of breast cancer, for which the 5-year relative survival rate following diagnosis is now more than 80% (CIHI and Statistics Canada, 2001). Among men, lung cancer, which is more often fatal, is wider spread.

Diabetes was also responsible for huge losses of autonomy. Among men, there was an 10.7 year difference in disability-free life expectancy between those with diabetes and those without. This difference rose to almost 14.1 years among women. The differential impact by sex on disability-free life expectancy was much less strong than for life expectancy. Songer (2001) showed that diabetes-related disabilities were more common among women than among men (in the total population), but the differences were not significant. The disabling effect of diabetes might thus be similar among both sexes, explaining the lower differences.

As expected, cancer had a major impact on mortality and a relatively minor impact on morbidity. Reducing male life expectancy by more than 11 years, cancer was the most fatal of the risk factors and chronic conditions considered here. The life expectancy of women with cancer was 12.9 years less than those without, ranking cancer just behind diabetes among these risk factors and chronic conditions. Generally, cancer cut off about one-third of the remaining life expectancy of both sexes. Its impact on mortality was so great that, at age 45, individuals with cancer could expect to live fewer years with disability than those without the disease. Consequently, elimination of cancer can be expected to result in a relative and absolute expansion of morbidity, due to the greater number of individuals reaching advanced ages at which disability becomes most prevalent.

Figure 1 summarizes the information in Table 3 and allows us to compare the differences in life expectancy and disability-free life ex-

FIGURE 1. Differences in Life Expectancy and Disability-Free Life Expectancy at 45 Years With versus Without Selected Risk Factors and Chronic Conditions by Sex, Canada, 1995 (Multi-State Model)

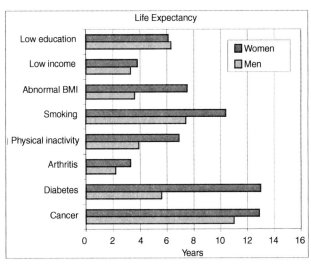

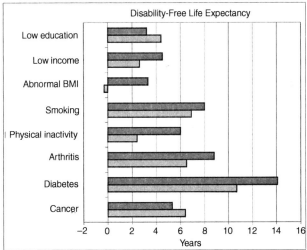

pectancy, by sex, according to the presence or absence of risk factors and chronic conditions. In general, chronic conditions had greater effects than socioeconomic and behavioural risk factors on both mortality and morbidity. Among the affected women, diabetes, cancer, and smoking were responsible for the biggest losses of life expectancy. Among men, cancer took first place, followed by smoking and then low education and diabetes. The well-known links between lung cancer and smoking certainly explain some of these results.

Diabetes, arthritis, and smoking were the risk factors and chronic conditions with the biggest impacts on disability-free life expectancy among affected women. Among affected men, the biggest impacts were from diabetes, smoking, cancer, and arthritis. For educational level and cancer, the loss of disability-free life expectancy was greater among men than women.

Table 4 presents the relative burden of disability, expressed as the proportion of life expectancy lived with or without disability, for each of the risk factors and chronic conditions. The proportion of years lived with disability was very high for individuals with diabetes. Not only were life expectancies of individuals with diabetes much shorter than those of others, but fewer of those years were lived disability-free. Consequently, the proportion of already shortened life expectancies likely to be disability-free was just 43% among diabetic men and 35% among diabetic women. No other risk factor or chronic condition had this kind of impact on affected individuals.

Among the risk factors and chronic conditions under study, arthritis had the least impact on the life expectancy of affected individuals (accounting for losses of 3.3 years for women, and 2.2 years for men). However, at age 45, 55% of the remaining life expectancy of women with arthritis was expected to be lived with disability, while the corresponding figure for men was 46%. For both men and women, then, the impact of arthritis on this indicator was second only to that of diabetes.

Individuals who did not smoke, like those at moderate or high income levels, could expect to live considerably more disability-free years compared to smokers and low income individuals. Non-smokers, in particular, could expect to live longer than smokers and to live disability-free longer, as well as to spend smaller proportions of their lives with disability.

Only slight changes in the proportion of life spent with disability were observed according to the presence or absence of low education, low income, physical inactivity, or abnormal body mass index.

Since cancer had a significantly greater effect on mortality than on morbidity, the elimination of this disease would result in an absolute

TABLE 4. Percentage of Remaining Life Expectancy (LE) at Age 45 to Be Lived Disability-Free (DFLE) and With Disability (DLE), for the Total Population and for Selected Risk Factors and Chronic Conditions, by Sex, Canada, 1995 (Multi-State Model)

Risk factor or chronic condition	Men			Women		
	LE	DFLE	DLE	LE	DFLE	DLE
Total Population	100.0	67.8	32.2	100.0	59.9	40.1
Education						
Lower education	100.0	67.3	32.7	100.0	59.4	40.6
Higher education	100.0	67.7	32.3	100.0	58.4	41.6
Income						
Low income	100.0	66.7	33.3	100.0	57.0	43.0
Middle or high income	100.0	67.9	32.1	100.0	63.2	36.8
Smoking						
Smoker	100.0	63.3	36.7	100.0	55.9	44.1
Non-smoker	100.0	69.6	30.4	100.0	61.3	38.7
Body Mass Index (BMI)						
Abnormal BMI	100.0	75.5	24.5	100.0	63.2	36.8
Normal BMI	100.0	66.6	33.4	100.0	59.6	40.4
Physical Activity						
Inactive	100.0	69.0	31.0	100.0	58.9	41.1
Active	100.0	68.2	31.8	100.0	63.3	36.7
Arthritis						
Yes	100.0	53.7	46.3	100.0	44.6	55.4
No	100.0	69.7	30.3	100.0	63.6	36.4
Diabetes						
Yes	100.0	43.3	56.7	100.0	35.4	64.6
No	100.0	68.2	31.8	100.0	59.7	40.3
Cancer						
Yes	100.0	71.3	28.7	100.0	68.2	31.8
No	100.0	67.1	32.9	100.0	59.2	40.8

and relative expansion of morbidity. This is because the number of additional years of life expectancy for individuals without cancer was so high and they were thus more likely to have disabilities, which are more common late in life. For individuals with cancer, the disease often resulted in a relatively quick death, and while a certain period of disability may be experienced, it was probably shorter than for other diseases.

DISCUSSION

An incidence-based multi-state life table method was used to generate estimates of life expectancies and disability-free life expectancies according to various health risk factors and chronic conditions. This exercise was aimed at showing how the elimination, or more realistically the reduction, of these factors would improve the health of the affected individuals. The impact of each risk factor was, however, assessed separately from each of the others. In each instance, the population was split into two groups: one with and one without the risk factor or chronic condition, based on the answers given by respondents to the survey. For this reason, our results for particular risk factors and chronic conditions are not additive across the factors or conditions. In contrast with Mathers (1992) and Nusselder (1998), who use methods which consider confounding and interactions between risk factors and chronic conditions, relative gains in life expectancy reported here must be considered in the context of, but independent of, other diseases.

Similarly, the impact of each risk factor or chronic condition on mortality and morbidity was measured independently of the other factors: no control variables were introduced into the models except age, sex, and functional state. In fact, many studies have shown links between these factors, for instance, smokers tend to be less active, less educated and have lower incomes than non-smokers, as well as generally strong links between diabetes and heart disease. Failing to take these relationships into account could produce an overestimate of the impact of diabetes or any other factor on mortality and morbidity. A set of nested models were produced to assess the stability of the estimators when different control variables were introduced in turn; in most cases the regression coefficients remained stable. This suggests that, statistically, the assumption of interdependence of the risk factors and chronic conditions has been verified and should not have skewed the results.

This method also did not permit a simple estimate to be made of uncertainty indicators such as standard errors and confidence intervals. Observed differences should thus be carefully interpreted when they are small. Use of micro-simulation based models will soon permit such indicators to be produced.

For use in establishing health policies at the population level, the calculation of potential gains due to the elimination of a given risk factor or chronic condition must also take into consideration the prevalence of the risk factor or chronic condition in the population as a whole. Our study showed that diabetes was the chronic disease with the greatest impact by far on both life expectancy and disability-free life expectancy of affected individuals. However, this disease only affected a small portion of the Canadian population (less than 10%), thereby limiting the impact of a program designed to eliminate diabetes (Table 5). Thus, to calculate the public health impacts at the population level, the results for the group without the risk factor or chronic condition should be com-

TABLE 5. Life Expectancy (LE), Disability-Free Life Expectancy (DFLE), and Disabled Life Expectancy (DLE) at Age 45, With versus Without Selected Risk Factors and Chronic Conditions, by Sex, Canada, 1995: Impact on Affected Individuals and Impact on Population Health

Risk factor or chronic condition	Men				Women			
	LE	DFLE	DLE		LE	DFLE	DLE	
			Any	*Severe*			*Any*	*Severe*
Impact on affected individuals								
Low education	6.3	4.4	1.9	−0.3	6.1	3.2	3.5	−0.1
Low income	3.3	2.6	0.7	−1.3	3.8	4.5	−0.7	−1.9
Smoking	7.4	6.9	0.4	−0.0	10.4	8.0	2.4	0.7
Abnormal BMI	3.6	−0.3	3.9	0.0	7.5	3.3	4.0	0.3
Physical inactivity	3.9	2.4	1.5	−0.2	6.9	6.0	0.9	−0.7
Arthritis	2.2	6.5	−4.2	−0.4	3.3	8.8	−5.5	−0.2
Diabetes	5.6	10.7	−5.1	−10.0	13.0	14.1	−1.1	−0.9
Cancer	11.0	6.4	4.6	1.0	12.9	5.3	7.6	1.3
Impact on population health								
Low education	4.3	2.9	1.4	−0.3	4.6	2.1	2.7	−0.1
Low income	0.7	0.5	0.2	−0.3	−0.2	1.1	−1.3	−1.5
Smoking	2.6	2.4	0.1	0.0	3.1	2.4	0.7	0.2
Abnormal BMI	0.9	0.2	0.7	0.0	1.9	1.0	0.7	0.1
Physical inactivity	2.9	2.1	0.8	−0.5	5.9	5.0	0.9	−0.9
Arthritis	0.4	0.9	−0.5	0.1	1.0	2.0	−1.0	0.3
Diabetes	0.4	0.4	0.0	0.0	1.3	0.7	0.6	0.1
Cancer	1.1	0.5	0.6	0.2	1.3	0.5	0.8	0.4

Note: Impact on affected individuals defined as difference between the expectancy for those without the risk factor or chronic condition less the expectancy for those with the risk factor or chronic condition.
Impact on population health defined as difference between the expectancy for those without the risk factor or chronic condition less the expectancy for the total population.
DLE *Any* includes any disability or institutionalization; DLE *Severe* includes severe disability or institutionalization.

pared with the results for the population as a whole. For instance, while diabetes results in 13.0 years fewer years of life expectancy for women with the disease, the elimination of the disease would result in an increase of only 1.3 years of life expectancy for the female population as a whole. Among men, the corresponding increase would be only 0.4 years. For disability-free life expectancy, the impact of diabetes on population health would be 0.4 and 0.7 additional years for men and women, respectively.

Under this same heading, the battle against smoking, a frequently fatal and disabling affliction, generates more hope, since almost 30% of the population were classified as smokers. The impact of programs aimed at getting people to cut back on smoking could have significant effects on average lifespan as well as on the quality of life of Canadian men and women. The elimination of smoking would result in an increase in remaining disability-free life expectancy at age 45 of 2.4 years for both men and women (Table 5). Smaller but substantial gains in disability-free life expectancy could result from programs aimed at reducing the prevalence of low-income (0.5 and 1.1 years, respectively, for men and women).

The battle against arthritis, the leading chronic health problem in Canada (Statistics Canada, 2001b), could also considerably increase disability-free life within the population, particularly in the case of women. Eliminating this rarely fatal disease would, however, contribute much less to extending average life expectancy. The elimination of cancer, a disease which is far less prevalent than the other chronic diseases examined here, would add little more than a year to the life expectancies of Canadian men and women, while adding only about half a year of disability-free life. By contrast, the population health impact of low education on disability-free life expectancy was estimated as 2.9 years for men, and 2.1 years for women. For physical inactivity, the corresponding impacts were estimated to be 2.1 years for men and 5.0 years for women.

It is difficult to establish the roots of gender inequality with respect to death and disease. We can, however, assess their impacts. Moreover, the indicators presented in this study are useful tools for decision makers seeking to define new strategies in the battles against various diseases or certain kinds of behaviour that are harmful to health. Up to now, much energy has been devoted to reducing the impact of fatal diseases like cancer. The calculation of disability-free life expectancies in the presence or absence of disease shows that in terms of population health, such policies would do relatively little to improve average life expectancy and even less to improve disability-free life expectancy. By contrast, decreases in chronic diseases like arthritis or diabetes and harmful behaviours like smoking, or reductions in physical inactivity and the prevalence of low education, could increase both the average life expectancy of the population and the average duration of disability-free life.

NOTES

1. However, we know this assumption is not always true. The increased efficacy of treatments for certain diseases can prolong survival, without actually improving quality of life. Life expectancy can thus rise, without general health conditions improving, resulting in an expansion of morbidity (Verbrugge, 1984; Olshansky et al., 1991).

2. Mathers' (1992) work on this subject was presented in a paper to the fifth meeting of the International Network on Health Expectancy (REVES) in Ottawa (Canada) in 1992.

3. This restriction was motivated by our use of activity limitations and dependency to define functional states. Very few individuals report such limitations or dependency before the age of 45.

4. This means sample size has gradually decreased with each cycle, but Statistics Canada recalculates the survey weights at each such cycle to take this factor into account along with cases of respondents who could not be located or who did not want to participate, in terms of a two-stage stratified design and post hoc stratification (Tambay et al., 1998). Attrition was relatively low, did not constitute a major source of bias, and did not considerably increase the variance estimates produced.

5. For men, the thresholds averaged about 22 and 31, while for women they averaged about 20 and 32.

6. The exact question was: "Do(es) . . . have any of the following long-term conditions that have been diagnosed by a health professional?"

7. In addition to the functional states and risk factors or chronic conditions under study, the model took into consideration age and an interaction variable between age and these states. The introduction of this interaction variable enabled the relative risks for the various functional states to converge as age increased. The assumption was that the functional state of a younger person would have a greater impact on his or her probability of dying than that of an older person

8. The CATMOD procedure in SAS.

9. This assumption was confirmed by the NPHS. Nearly two-thirds (65%) of women 45 years or older classified as non-smokers said they had never smoked, a proportion nearly double that of male non-smokers (35%).

REFERENCES

Bélanger, A. (1999). *Report on the Demographic Situation in Canada, 1998-1999.* Statistics Canada Catalogue 91-209-XPE. Ministry of Industry, Ottawa, 1999, Table A9, 109.

Bronnum-Hansen, H. and K. Juel. (2001). Abstention from smoking extends life and compresses morbidity: A population based study of health expectancy among smokers and never smokers in Denmark. *Tobacco Control*, 10, 3, 273-278.

Canadian Institute for Health Information (CIHI) and Statistics Canada. (2001). *Health Care in Canada.* Canadian Institute for Health Information, Ottawa.

Chen, J. and Millar, W. (2001). Starting and sustaining physical activity. *Health Reports* (Statistics Canada, catalogue 82-003), 12, 4, 33-43.

Doblhammer, G. and Kytir, J. (1998). Social inequalities in disability-free and healthy life expectancy in Austria. *Wien Klin Wochenschr,* 110, 11, 393-396.

Ferrucci, L., Izmirlian, G., Léveillé, S.G., Phillips, C.L., Corti, M.C., Brock, D.B., and Guralnik, J.M. (1999). Smoking, physical activity, and active life expectancy. *American Journal of Epidemiology,* 149, 7, 645-653.

Geiss, L.S., Herman, W. H., and Smith, P.J. (2001). Mortality in non-insulin-dependent diabetes. *Diabetes in America,* 2nd edition, http://diabetes-in-america.s-3.com. contents.htm, 233-257.

Giardina, E.G. (2000). Heart disease in women. *International Journal of Fertility and Women's Medicine,* 45, 6, 350-357.

Guralnik, J.M., Land, K.C., Blazer, D., Fillenbaum, G.C., and Branch, L.G. (1993). Educational state and active life expectancy among older blacks and whites. *New England Journal of Medicine,* 329, 2, 110-116.

Keller, K.B. and Lemberg, L. (2000). Gender differences in acute coronary events. *American Journal of Critical Care,* 9, 3, 207-209.

Laditka, J.N. and S.B. Laditka. (2001). Effects of diabetes on healthy life expectancy: Shorter lives with more disability for both women and men. Paper presented at IUSSP seminar on longer life and healthy aging, Beijing, October 22-24th.

Leigh, J.P. and Fries, J.F. (1994). Education, gender, and the compression of morbidity. *International Journal of Aging and Human Development,* 39, 3, 233-246.

Léveillé, S.G., Resnick, H.E., and Balfour, J. (2000). Gender differences in disability: Evidence and underlying reasons. *Aging,* 12, 2, 106-112.

Manton, K. G. (1997). Demographic trends for the aging female population. *Journal of the American Medical Women's Association,* 52, 3, 99-105.

Martel, L., Bélanger, A., and Berthelot, J.-M. (2000). Risk factors associated with the transitions between health states: Some results from longitudinal panel of NPHS. Paper presented at the REVES 12 Meeting, Healthy Life Expectancy: Linking Policy and Science, Los Angeles, March 20 to 22, 2000.

Mathers, C. (1992). Estimating gains in health expectancy due to elimination of specific diseases. Paper presented at the 5th meeting of the International Network on Health Expectancy (REVES-5), February 19-21, Ottawa, Canada.

Melzer, D., McWilliams, B., Brayne, C., Johnson, T., and Bond, J. (2000). Socioeconomic state and the expectation of disability in old age: Estimates for England. *Journal of Epidemiology and Community Health,* 54, 2, 286-292.

Millar, W. and Stephens, T. (1992). Social state and health risks in Canadian adults, 1985 and 1991. *Health Reports* (Statistics Canada, catalogue 82-003), 5, 143-156.

Nault, F., Roberge, R., and Berthelot, J.-M. (1996). Espérance de vie et espérance de vie en santé selon le sexe, l'état matrimonial et le statut socio-économique au Canada. *Cahiers Québécois de Démographie,* 25, 2, 241-259.

Nusselder, W.J. (1998). *Compression or Expansion of Morbidity? A Life-table Approach.* Thesis Publishers, Amsterdam, 253 pp.

Olshansky, S.J., Rudberg, M.A., Carnes, B.A., Cassel, C.K., and Brody, J.A. (1991). Trading off longer life for worsening health. *Journal of Aging and Health*, 3, 2, 194-216.

Prescott, E.I., Osler, M. Hein, H.O., Borch-Johnsen, K., Schnohr, P., and Vestbo, J. (1999). Smoking and life expectancy among Danish men and women. *Ugeskr Laeger*, 161, 9, 1261-1263.

Rogers, RG., Nam, C.B., and Hummer, R.A. (1994). Activity limitations and cigarette smoking in the United States: Implications for health expectancies. In *Advances in Health Expectancies*, C.D. Mathers, J. McCallum and J.-M. Robine (eds.), Canberra, Australian Institute of Health and Welfare, 337-344.

Songer, T. J. (2001). Disability in diabetes. *Diabetes in America*, 2nd edition, http://diabetes-in-america.s-3.com.contents.htm, 259-282.

Statistics Canada. (2000). Women in Canada 2000: A gender-based statistical report. *Statistics Canada Target Groups Project*, catalogue 89-503, Minister of Industry, Ottawa, 49-88.

Statistics Canada. (2001a). *Report on the demographic situation in Canada 2000*. Catalogue 91-209, Minister of Industry, Ottawa, 203 pp.

Statistics Canada (2001b). How healthy are Canadians? *Health Reports* (catalogue 82-003), 12, 3, special issue.

Tambay, J.-L., Schiopu-Kratina, I., Mayda, J., Stukel, D., and Nadon, S. (1998). Treatment of nonresponse in Cycle Two of the National Population Health Survey. *Survey Methodology* (Statistics Canada, catalogue 12-001), 24, 2, 147-156.

Valkonen, T., Sihvonen, A.P., and Lahelma, E. (1997). Health expectancy by level of education in Finland. *Social Science and Medicine*, 44, 6, 801-808.

Verbrugge, L.M. (1984). Longer life but worsening health? Trends in health and mortality of middle-aged and older persons. *Milbank Memorial Fund Quarterly/Health and Society*, 62, 3, 475-519.

WHO (World Health Organization) (1995). Physical state: The use and interpretation of anthropometry. Report of the WHO Expert Committee, *WHO Technical Report Series*, no. 854, Geneva.

Wigle, D.T. (1995). Canada's health state: A public health perspective. *Risk Analysis*, 15, 6, 693-698.

Gender Differences in Life Expectancy Free of Impairment at Older Ages

Carol Jagger, PhD
Fiona Matthews, MSc

SUMMARY. This article uses data from the United Kingdom Medical Research Council Cognitive Function and Ageing study (MRC CFAS) to analyze morbidity associated with three areas of impairment. We use cognitive status, functional status, and physical illness to examine differences in the proportion of time that older women and men will spend with co-morbidity. We also analyze differences among various impair-

Carol Jagger is Professor of Epidemiology in the Department of Epidemiology and Public Health at the University of Leicester.

Fiona Matthews is the statistician for the Cognitive Function and Ageing Study and is affiliated with the Medical Research Council Biostatistics Unit in Cambridge.

To review the Medical Research Council Cognitive Function and Ageing Study see *www. mrc-bsu.cam.ac.uk/cfas* for details of collaborators.

Address correspondence to: Fiona Matthews, MRC Biostatistics Unit, Institute of Public Health, University Forvie Site, Robinson Way, Cambridge CB2 2SR, England (E-mail: *fiona.matthews@mrc-bsu.cam.ac.uk*).

MRC CFAS is supported by major awards from the Medical Research Council and the Department of Health. The authors appreciate the cooperation of the Family Health Service Authorities of each centre, in providing the appropriate lists of patients, and in helping trace those who move within and outside the areas. The authors are indebted to the local general practitioners and their staff for the support and assistance. The authors warmly thank the interviewers for their heroic efforts, and volunteers who allowed us to practice on them. Thanks are especially due to the residents of East Cambridgeshire, Liverpool, Ynys Mon, Dwyfor, Newcastle upon Tyne, Nottingham, and Oxford for their continuing participation in the study.

[Haworth co-indexing entry note]: "Gender Differences in Life Expectancy Free of Impairment at Older Ages." Jagger, Carol, and Fiona Matthews. Co-published simultaneously in *Journal of Women & Aging* (The Haworth Press, Inc.) Vol. 14, No. 1/2, 2002, pp. 85-97; and: *Health Expectations for Older Women: International Perspectives* (ed: Sarah B. Laditka) The Haworth Press, Inc., 2002, pp. 85-97. Single or multiple copies of this article are available for a fee from The Haworth Document Delivery Service [1-800-HAWORTH 9:00 a.m. - 5:00 p.m. (EST). E-mail address: getinfo@haworthpressinc.com].

85

ments, and investigate the relationship between missing data and sex. Women have a larger burden of impairment than men, and, by including cognitive impairment together with functional impairment, a very large impairment burden is highlighted at all ages. Policy implications of the findings from the perspective of older women in the United Kingdom are discussed. *[Article copies available for a fee from The Haworth Document Delivery Service: 1-800-HAWORTH. E-mail address: <getinfo@haworthpressinc. com> Website: <http://www.HaworthPress.com> © 2002 by The Haworth Press, Inc. All rights reserved.]*

KEYWORDS. Cognitive impairment, functional status, missing data, health expectancy

INTRODUCTION

The process of disablement with ageing has tended to be focussed at the point where there is an impact on the daily life activities of older people, the so-called Activities of Daily Living (ADLs) (Katz, Ford, Moskowitz, Jackson, and Jaffe, 1963) based on personal care items and Instrumental Activities of Daily Living (IADLs) which are concerned with household level activities such as shopping and cooking (Lawton and Brody, 1969). There have been a number of major models of the disablement process (Nagi, 1965; Wood, 1975; World Health Organization, 1980; Nagi, 1991; Verbrugge and Jette, 1994) with each distinguishing between a maximum of five states: disease; impairments; functional limitations; activity restriction; and handicap, the major differences being in distinguishing states later in the sequence and particularly the distinction between functional limitations and activity restriction. A key point is that all these models agree on the position of diseases and impairments on the disablement process. Nagi (1965) defined impairments as anatomical, physiological, intellectual or emotional abnormalities, or losses and noted that, despite their position in the process after disease, impairments do not always imply a disease in the sense of active pathology.

Impairments are thus an important stage in the disablement process and older ages are often characterized by the higher prevalence of these, particularly cognitive impairments. Women tend to exhibit a higher prevalence of cognitive impairments than men. As the evidence for differences in incidence are less strong (Fratiglioni et al., 2000), this may in part be due to their longer survival with dementia (Jagger, Clarke, and Stone, 1995).

The area of mental health expectancy has received less attention than health expectancies based on measures of physical function, usually disability based on ADL restrictions, and has tended to be centred around disease, in terms of dementia-free life expectancy (Ritchie, Robine, Letenneur, and Dartigues, 1994; Jagger et al., 1998; Sauvaget, Tsuji, Haan, and Hisamichi, 1999). We present data from a very large multi-centre study to examine the differential time spent with cognitive and functional impairments and with physical illness between women and men in the United Kingdom. A previous paper (MRC CFAS, 2001) presented each type of impairment and the burden on the population but an important problem in such studies of cognitive impairment, and indeed of almost all studies of the very old, is that of non-response or response by a proxy, which results in larger quantities of missing data. Impairment in one dimension may influence missing data in another dimension and hence we also investigate the degree to which the current estimates of the impairment burden are influenced by differential amounts of missing data by sex within the impairments investigated.

METHODS

The MRC Cognitive Function and Ageing study (MRC CFAS) is a multi-centre prospective cohort study. Set up in 1989 by the Medical Research Council (MRC) and the Department of Health (DoH), its aim is to study ageing, cognitive function, and dementia across England and Wales. The core study had five methodologically similar centres (Cambridgeshire, Gwynedd, Newcastle, Nottingham, Oxford) and one centre (Liverpool) that was funded earlier but has a slightly different design. The five centres selected a stratified random sample from Family Health Service Authority lists of sufficient individuals aged 65 years and over to achieve at least 2,500 interviews at each centre. Respondents were screened with a basic interview and approximately 20% were selected on the basis of age and cognitive performance to receive a more detailed clinically orientated assessment interview one to two months later. This paper uses data from the five methodologically similar centres with a total sample size of 13,009 adults aged 65 years and over (data version 3.1); full details have already been reported (MRC CFAS, 1998).

Respondents were interviewed in their homes using laptop computers with immediate entry of response codes about marital status, accommodation, occupation (for social class), social networks (Wenger, 1989), ADLs (Bond and Carstairs, 1982), cognitive function (Folstein, Folstein, and McHugh, 1975; MRC, 1987), the organicity section questions from the Geriatric Mental State Examination (Copeland, Dewy, and Griffiths-Jones, 1986), medication and physical health questions relevant to dementia and cognitive health (Launer, Brayne, and Breteler, 1992). Signed informed consent was obtained from the respondent or from a proxy where appropriate.

Three types of impairment are considered: functional, based on the Townsend disability scale (maximum 18 points) with a cut point of 11 or above indicating functional impairment and equating to standard methods (Townsend, 1979); cognitive impairment, defined as a score below 18 on the Mini-Mental State Examination (MMSE) (Brayne and Calloway, 1990); and physical impairment, taken as being the presence of any of the conditions (stroke, heart attack, angina, high blood pressure, peripheral vascular disease, transient ischaemic attacks, severe hearing or visual problems, epilepsy, asthma [except childhood only], chronic bronchitis, Parkinson's disease, depression, and arthritis).

The interview was designed so that in cases of severe cognitive impairment, or where the interviewer considered the respondent was not able to answer the entire interview, a subset of questions could be asked; this decision could be made at any time by either the interviewer, the proxy, or the respondent. In this "priority interview," questions concentrated on cognition and did not include functional impairment or health. Proxy interviews were also permitted for all sections, except cognition, which would therefore be missing in these instances.

Statistical Methods

The proportion of individuals in each age and sex group were tabulated as suffering from none, one, two, or all three of these impairment dimensions. People with missing values were those who had already reached the threshold for impairment, or where the threshold could not be crossed regardless of the possible responses to the missing data. Health expectancies were then calculated combining the prevalence with mortality data (OPCS, 1993) using the Sullivan method (Sullivan, 1971), and with life expectancies calculated up to the age of 90 years in single years of age. Those with missing data were included as impaired in one analysis to investigate the extent to which gender differences found could be explained by differential amounts of missing information.

RESULTS

A total of 7,849 women and 5,160 men had the basic screening interview that provided information on the three areas of impairment. Table 1 shows the prevalence of the three impairments by five-year age group and the degree of missing data. Below 80 years of age, women exhibited greater rates of physical and functional impairment than men but similar levels of cognitive impairment. Missing data was relatively rare in these age groups. Rates of cognitive and functional impairment rose with age for both sexes and after age 80 women had substantially higher rates than men. The relationship between age and physical impairment was less clear with older women having very similar levels of physical impairment to men of the same age. Missing data for each impairment increased with age with a tendency for there to be more missing data for women than men in each age group. The remaining life expectancy for women was almost four years more than for men in the youngest age group (65-69 years) decreasing to 0.6 years in the highest age group (90+ years) (Table 1).

TABLE 1. Percentage of the Study Population With Each of the Three Impairment Types, Together With the Percentage That Had Missing Data for That Impairment (in Parentheses) by Age and Sex

	Age	No.	Cognitive impairment		Functional impairment		Physical impairment		Life expectancy
Women	**65-69**	1,743	1	(<1)	5	(<1)	84	(<1)	17.8
	70-74	1,763	2	(<1)	5	(<1)	85	(<1)	14.2
	75-79	1,748	2	(1)	11	(2)	86	(2)	10.9
	80-84	1,477	11	(3)	22	(7)	85	(5)	8.0
	85-89	792	19	(5)	33	(11)	84	(7)	5.7
	90+	326	37	(10)	46	(24)	81	(13)	3.9
Men	**65-69**	1,444	1	(<1)	3	(<1)	80	(<1)	14.1
	70-74	1,386	2	(<1)	4	(1)	81	(1)	11.0
	75-79	1,160	4	(<1)	8	(2)	85	(1)	8.4
	80-84	778	5	(2)	12	(2)	86	(2)	6.3
	85-89	302	14	(3)	19	(9)	83	(5)	4.6
	90+	90	18	(3)	38	(14)	80	(6)	3.3

Impairment combinations are shown in Table 2. Physical impairment was both the most common single impairment, and together with functional impairment, the most common shared impairment combination. Physical impairment alone was the most common condition in both sexes and at all ages, except in women aged 90+ where physical impairment and functional impairment was equally common (28% compared with 30% respectively). Since by definition the row percentages in Table 2 sum to 100%, including the missing data as impaired resulted in changes across all the impairment combinations and had the most effect at the oldest ages and with three impairment combinations. These results were similar in both men and women with the pattern of impairment combinations remaining substantially the same whether the missing data was excluded or included. However, excluding the missing data suggests that the impairment burden could be underestimated, particularly in women and in the oldest age groups.

When all those with missing information and not already deemed impaired were excluded, women appear to spend more absolute years and a longer proportion of their remaining life with impairments than men (Figure 1). For example a 70-year-old woman had a total life expectancy of 14.2 years with 1.6 years with no impairment (11%), 9.9 years with one impairment (70%), 2.3 years with two impairments (16%), and 0.5 years with three impairments (3%). By age 85 years, women could expect to spend 11% of remaining life impaired physically, functionally, and cognitively compared to 4% of the remaining life for men. Including those with missing data as impaired increased these figures for both men and women (to 25% for women and 15% for men), but had negligible effect on the gender differential (Figure 2).

DISCUSSION

This study clearly shows the impact of cognitive, functional, and physical impairments on older men and women with women spending a greater proportion of their remaining life with impairment. A major problem faced by studies of ageing are the increasing levels of cognitive impairment with age, often resulting in significant amounts of missing data for other self-report measures. In general, this is dealt with in analyses by reporting comparisons of those with missing data and those without on broad demographic characteristics, such as age and sex and then excluding those with missing data in subsequent analyses. Because of the nature of our study, missing data was predominantly due to im-

TABLE 2. Percentage of the Study Population by Each Impairment Combination by Age and Sex, Missing Excluded and Missing Included as Impaired (in Parentheses)[1]

		None	Physical	Functional	Cognitive	Physical & Functional	Physical & Cognitive	Functional & Cognitive	All three
Women	65-69	29 (29)	66 (65)	<1 (<1)	<1 (<1)	4 (4)	<1 (1)	0 (<1)	<1 (1)
	70-74	26 (26)	68 (67)	1 (1)	<1 (<1)	4 (5)	1 (1)	<1 (<1)	<1 (1)
	75-79	24 (24)	63 (62)	1 (1)	<1 (1)	10 (10)	1 (1)	<1 (<1)	1 (3)
	80-84	19 (18)	54 (50)	2 (2)	1 (1)	17 (17)	2 (3)	1 (1)	3 (10)
	85-89	13 (11)	45 (39)	2 (2)	2 (2)	26 (24)	5 (5)	1 (1)	6 (16)
	90+	8 (6)	28 (20)	7 (5)	1 (1)	30 (23)	5 (4)	3 (3)	18 (39)
Men	65-69	29 (29)	67 (67)	<1 (<1)	<1 (<1)	3 (3)	<1 (<1)	0 (<1)	<1 (1)
	70-74	28 (27)	67 (66)	<1 (<1)	<1 (<1)	4 (4)	1 (1)	0 (0)	<1 (1)
	75-79	23 (22)	67 (65)	1 (1)	1 (1)	6 (7)	1 (1)	0 (0)	1 (3)
	80-84	19 (19)	67 (64)	1 (1)	1 (1)	10 (10)	2 (2)	0 (0)	1 (4)
	85-89	18 (16)	58 (52)	1 (2)	1 (1)	15 (14)	3 (3)	1 (1)	3 (12)
	90+	15 (12)	41 (34)	5 (4)	0 (0)	29 (28)	1 (1)	0 (0)	8 (20)

[1]Within sex and age group, row percentages for missing excluded sum to 100 as do those for missing included as impaired (percentages in parentheses).

FIGURE 1. Percentage of Total Life Expectancy With Number of Impairments, by Age and Sex, Missing Data Excluded

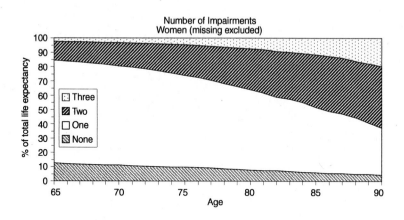

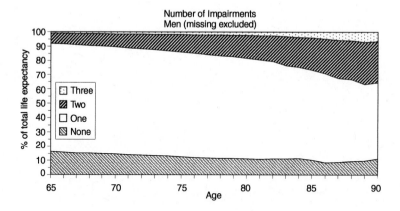

paired cognitive function, with greater amounts of missing data for women compared to men of the same age. Comparison of the effect of excluding those with missing data with including them as impaired showed that the gender differentials in the proportion of life expectancy with impairment were relatively unaffected and, therefore, were not a result of differential amounts of missing data between men and women.

FIGURE 2. Percentage of Total Life Expectancy With Number of Impairments, by Age and Sex, Missing Data Included as Impaired

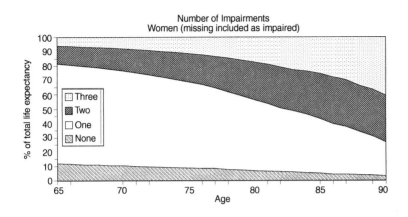

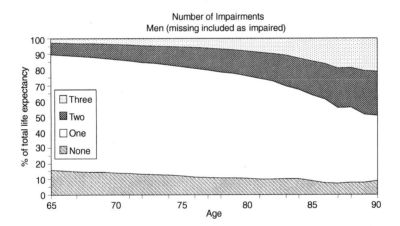

To date, health expectancies have tended to focus on physical health measures such as disability-free life expectancies with many fewer studies reporting health expectancies based on measures of mental health or indeed on combinations of impairments as reported here. Estimates of life expectancy spent with dementia appear to be similar from studies across Europe and relatively static with age, at around one year for women and half a year for men (Jagger et al., 1998). However, most of the studies reported have included relatively few of the very old (aged 90 years and over) and hence it is difficult to predict whether these estimates remain static over the entire age range. The only comparable study, from Melton Mowbray, England (Jagger et al., 1991), reported life expectancy with cognitive impairment, using the MMSE with a cut point of 24 and scoring those unable to answer as impaired on each item of the MMSE. Despite the less severe levels of cognitive impairment detected, women again showed significantly greater proportions of remaining life spent with cognitive impairment (Bone et al., 1995). Measures of physical and functional impairment in the Melton Mowbray study were, however, not directly comparable with MRC CFAS.

The measures used here had different sensitivities to the impairment types. Physical impairment was the presence of one of many self-reported conditions and hence current physical disability cannot be assumed. Cognitive and functional impairments were considered on a cut-point of a well-used ordinal scale measured at the time of interview. No severity information could be incorporated for the physical impairment to attempt to address this discrepancy; however, severity could be examined for both functional and cognitive impairment.

We found all three impairments to be more common in women than in men, consistent with other studies (e.g., Ferrucci et al., 1999; Crimmins, Hayward, and Saito, 1996; Tsuji et al., 1995). These findings have important policy implications since, as women are more likely to be widowed and live alone than are men, the bulk of the care needs falls to children, neighbours, and the formal health and social care services. This is more problematic when the woman is cognitively impaired since care needs are not as predictable and there is a greater likelihood of a move into residential care. Moreover, the strong relationship between the prevalence of cognitive impairment and age means that, as life expectancies continue to increase, the numbers of women with cognitive impairment will increase.

A further effect of the higher prevalence of cognitive impairment in women over men was that women had a larger amount of missing data. However, including the missing data as impaired changed the gender differences only marginally but had a considerable effect on the proportion of life spent with impairments for women and men. In most studies, missing data is not usually included and this could underestimate effects, particularly in the women. Our findings suggest that using studies where considerations of missing data have not been made, to project future health and care needs, would result in considerable underestimates of the burden on services with major implications for health planners and policy-makers.

Including measures of cognitive impairment into active life expectancy has been shown to significantly decrease estimates of active life expectancy by 6.8% in men aged 65 years and 10.1% in women (Gallo, Schoen, and Jones, 2000). Cognitive impairment has been shown to be an important precursor to the subsequent development of activity restriction in older people (Wood, 1975; Moritz, Kasl, and Berkman, 1995). Thus, combining measures of earlier and later stages in the disablement process will simply reflect the greater range of severity detected. Keeping the measures separate and estimating health expectancies based on each stage of the disablement process will instead help to elucidate scenarios like that of dynamic equilibrium (Manton, 1982). In this case, trends in disability of all levels remains static, though this hides increases in less severe disability over time together with falls in the more severe levels of disability. In addition, further longitudinal data to establish how impairments impact on the disablement process, particularly on social functioning and the need for care will provide a better picture of the future needs of older men and women in our populations and the relationship between this process and death.

REFERENCES

Bond, J., & Carstairs, V. (1982). *Services for the elderly.* Scottish Health Service Studies, No 42. Edinburgh: Scottish Home and Health Department.

Bone, M. R., Bebbington, A. C., Jagger, C., Morgan, K., & Nicolaas, G. (1995). *Health Expectancy and Its Uses.* London: HMSO.

Brayne, C., & Calloway, P. (1990). The case identification of dementia in the community: A comparison of methods. *International Journal of Geriatric Psychiatry*, 5, 309-316.

Copeland, J. R. M., Dewey, M. E., & Griffiths-Jones, H. M. (1986). A computerized psychiatric diagnostic system and case nomenclature for elderly subjects: GMS and AGECAT. *Psychological Medicine*, 16, 89-99.

Crimmins, E. M., Hayward, M. D., & Saito, Y. (1996). Differentials in active life expectancy in the older population of the United States. *Journal of Gerontology: Social Sciences*, 51B(3), S111-S120.

Ferrucci, L., Izmirlian, G., Leveille, S., Phillips, C. L., Corti, M. C., Brock, D. B., & Guralnick, J. M. (1999). Smoking, physical activity and active life expectancy. *American Journal of Epidemiology*, 149, 645-653.

Folstein, M. F., Folstein, S. E., & McHugh, P. R. (1975). Mini-mental state: A practical method for grading the cognitive state of patients for the clinician. *Journal of Psychiatric Research*, 313, 1419-1420.

Fratiglioni, L., Launer, L. J., Andersen, K., Breteler, M. M., Copeland, J. R., & Dartigues, J. F. et al. (2000). Incidence of dementia and major subtypes in Europe: A collaborative study of population-based cohorts. Neurologic Diseases in the Elderly Research Group. *Neurology*, 54, S10-S15.

Gallo, J. J., Schoen, R., & Jones, R. (2000). Cognitive impairment and syndromal depression in estimates of active life expectancy: The 13-year follow-up of the Baltimore Epidemiologic Catchment Area sample. *Acta Psychiatrica Scandinavica*, 101, 265-273.

Jagger, C., Clarke, M., & Clarke, S. J. (1991). Getting older feeling younger: The changing health profile of the elderly. *International Journal of Epidemiology*, 20, 234-238.

Jagger, C., Clarke, M., & Stone, A. (1995). Predictors of survival with Alzheimer's disease: A community-based study. *Psychological Medicine*, 25, 171-177.

Jagger, C., Ritchie, K., & Bronnun-Hansen, H. et al. (1998). Mental Health Expectancy: The European perspective. A synopsis of results presented at the Conference of the European Network for the Calculation of Health Expectancies (Euro-REVES). *Acta Psychiatrica Scandinavica*, 98, 85-91.

Katz, S., Ford, A. B., Moskowitz, R. W., Jackson, B. A., & Jaffe, M. W. (1963). Studies of illness in the aged. The Index of ADL: A standardized measure of biological and psychosocial function. *Journal of the American Medical Association*, 185, 914-919.

Launer, L. J., Brayne, C., & Breteler, M. M. B. (1992). Epidemiologic approach to the study of dementing diseases: A nested case-control study in European incidence studies of dementia. *Neuroepidemiology*, 11(1), 114-118.

Lawrence, R. H., & Jette, A. M. (1998). Disentangling the disablement process. *Journal of Gerontology: Social Sciences*, 51B(4), S173-S182.

Lawton, M. P., & Brody, E. M. (1969). Assessment of older people: Self-maintaining and instrumental activities of daily living. *The Gerontologist*, 9, 179-186.

Manton, K. G. (1982). Changing concepts of morbidity and mortality in the elderly population. *Milbank Memorial Fund Quarterly / Health and Society*, 60, 183-244.

Medical Research Council. (1987). *Report from the MRC Alzheimer's disease workshop*. London: Medical Research Council.

Moritz, D. J., Kasl, S. V., & Berkman, L. F. (1995). Cognitive functioning and the incidence of limitations in activities of daily living in an elderly community sample. *American Journal of Epidemiology*, 141, 41-49.

MRC CFAS. (1998). Cognitive function and dementia in six areas of England and Wales: The distribution of MMSE and prevalence of GMS organicity level in the MRC-CFA Study. *Psychological Medicine*, 28, 319-335.

MRC CFAS. (2001). Health and ill-health in the older population in England and Wales. *Age and Ageing*, 30, 53-62.

Nagi, S. Z. (1965). Some conceptual issues in disability and rehabilitation. In M. B. Sussman (Ed.), *Sociology and Rehabilitation*. Washington, DC: American Sociological Association.

Nagi, S. Z. (1991). Disability concepts revisited: Implication for prevention. In A.M. Pope, & A.R. Tatlov (Eds.), *Disability in America: Toward a national agenda for prevention*. Appendix A. Washington, DC: National Academy Press.

OPCS. (1993). *Mortality statistics–Series DH1 no 26.* London: HMSO.

Ritchie, K., Robine, J. M., Letenneur, L., & Dartigues, J. F. (1994). Dementia-free life expectancy in France. *American Journal of Public Health,* 84, 232-236.

Sauvaget, C., Tsuji, I., Haan, M. N., & Hisamichi, S. (1999). Trends in dementia-free life expectancy among elderly members of a large health maintenance organization. *International Journal of Epidemiology,* 28, 1110-1118.

Sullivan, D. F. (1971). A single index of mortality and morbidity. *HSMHA Health Reports,* 86, 347-354.

Townsend, P. (1979). *Poverty in the United Kingdom.* Harmondsworth: Pelican.

Tsuji, I., Minami, Y., Fukao, A., Hisamichi, S., Asano, H., & Sato, M. (1995). Active life expectancy among elderly Japanese. *Journal of Gerontology: Medical Sciences,* 50A, M173-M176.

Verbrugge, L. M., & Jette, A. M. (1994). The disablement process. *Social Science and Medicine,* 38, 1-14.

Wenger, G. C. (1989). Support networks in old age–constructing a typology. In M. Jeffreys (Ed.), *Growing old in the 20th century.* London: Routledge.

Wood, P. H. N. (1975). *Classification of impairments and handicaps.* World Health Organization (WHO/ICD 9/REV. CONF/75.15).

World Health Organization. (1980). *International Classification of Impairments, Disabilities, and Handicaps.* Geneva: World Health Organization (Reprint, 1993).

Global Patterns
of Healthy Life Expectancy
for Older Women

Colin D. Mathers, PhD
Christopher J. L. Murray, MD
Alan D. Lopez, PhD
Ritu Sadana, PhD
Joshua A. Salomon, PhD

SUMMARY. This paper focuses on patterns of healthy life expectancy for older women around the globe in the year 2000, and on the determinants of differences in disease and injury for older ages. Our study uses data from the World Health Organization for women and men in 191 countries. These data include a summary measure of population health, healthy life expectancy (HALE), which measures the number of years of life expected to be lived in good health, and a complementary measure of the loss of health (disability-adjusted life years or DALYs) due to a com-

Colin D. Mathers, Christopher J. L. Murray, Alan D. Lopez, Ritu Sadana, and Joshua A. Salomon are affiliated with the Global Programme on Evidence for Health Policy, World Health Organization, Geneva, Switzerland.

Address correspondence to: Dr. Colin D. Mathers, World Health Organization, Avenue Appia, 1211 Geneva 27, Switzerland (E-mail: mathersc@who.int).

The authors thank the many staff of the Global Program on Evidence for Health Policy who contributed to the development of life tables, burden of disease analysis and the development and conduct of the health surveys. These include Omar Ahmad, Lydia Bendib, Somnath Chatterji, Mie Inoue, Rafael Lozano, Doris Ma Fat, Claudia Stein, Bedirhan Ustun, and Cao Yang.

[Haworth co-indexing entry note]: "Global Patterns of Healthy Life Expectancy for Older Women." Mathers et al. Co-published simultaneously in *Journal of Women & Aging* (The Haworth Press, Inc.) Vol. 14, No. 1/2, 2002, pp. 99-117; and: *Health Expectations for Older Women: International Perspectives* (ed: Sarah B. Laditka) The Haworth Press, Inc., 2002, pp. 99-117. Single or multiple copies of this article are available for a fee from The Haworth Document Delivery Service [1-800-HAWORTH 9:00 a.m. - 5:00 p.m. (EST). E-mail address: getinfo@haworthpressinc.com].

prehensive set of disease and injury causes. We examine two topics in detail: (1) cross-national patterns of female-male differences in healthy life expectancy at age 60; and (2) identification of the major injury and disability causes of disability in women at older ages. Globally, the male-female gap is lower for HALE than for total life expectancy. The sex gap is highest for Russia (10.0 years) and lowest in North Africa and the Middle East, where males and females have similar levels of healthy life expectancy, and in some cases, females have lower levels of healthy life expectancy. We discuss the implications of the findings for international health policy. *[Article copies available for a fee from The Haworth Document Delivery Service: 1-800-HAWORTH. E-mail address: <getinfo@ haworthpressinc.com> Website: <http://www.HaworthPress.com> © 2002 by The Haworth Press, Inc. All rights reserved.]*

KEYWORDS. Older women, HALE, healthy life expectancy, health-adjusted life expectancy, DALE, compression of morbidity

INTRODUCTION

For the first time ever in its World Health Report 2000, the World Health Organization (WHO) reported on the average levels of population health for its 191 member countries using a summary measure that combines information on mortality and disability (WHO, 2000). The primary summary measure of population health used was Disability-Adjusted Life Expectancy, or DALE, which measures the equivalent number of years of life expected to be lived in full health (Mathers, Sadana et al., 2001). In the following year, updated estimates of healthy life expectancy for the year 2000 were published in the World Health Report 2001 (WHO, 2001) using improved methods and incorporating cross-population comparable survey data from 63 surveys in 55 countries. To better reflect the inclusion of all states of health in the calculation of healthy life expectancy, the name of the indicator used to measure healthy life expectancy was changed from disability-adjusted life expectancy (DALE) to healthy life expectancy (HALE).

In the last two decades, considerable international effort has been put into the development of summary measures of population health that integrate information of mortality and non-fatal health outcomes (Murray et al., 2001) and this special volume is another indication of the growing international policy interest in such indicators. There are two main classes of summary measures: health gaps and health expectancies. The Disability-Adjusted Life Year (DALY) is the best known health gap measure and quantifies the gap between a population's actual health and some defined goal (Murray & Lopez, 1996). HALE belongs to the family of health expectancies, summarizing the total life expectancy into equivalent years of "full health" by taking into account the distribution of health states (disability) in the population. WHO has chosen to use HALE as a summary measure of level of population health because it is relatively easy to explain the concept of an equivalent "healthy" life expectancy and because it is measured in units (years of life) that are meaningful to non-technical audiences (unlike other indicators, such as mortality rates or incidence rates).

HALE is also preferable as a summary measure of population to indicators such as Disability-Free Life Expectancy (DFLE) which incorporate a dichotomous weighting scheme. Because time spent in any health state categorized as disabled is assigned arbitrarily a weight of zero (equivalent to death), DFLE is not sensitive to differences in the severity distribution of disability in populations. In contrast, HALE adds up expectation of life for different health states with adjustment for severity distribution.

DFLE estimates based on self-reported health status information are not comparable across countries due to differences in survey instruments and cultural differences in reporting of health (Robine, Mathers, & Brouard, 1996). Analyses of over 50 national health surveys for the calculation of healthy life expectancy in the World Health Report 2000 identified severe limitations in the comparability of self-report health status data from different populations, even when identical survey instruments and methods were used (Sadana et al., 2000). We have demonstrated how these comparability problems relate not only to differences in survey design and methods, but much more fundamentally to unmeasured differences in expectations and norms for health. For example, the cutpoints of scales for a given domain such as mobility may have very different meanings across different cultures, across socio-economic groups within a society, across age groups or between men and women (Sadana et al., 2000; Murray et al., 2000). During the last two years, WHO has embarked on large-scale efforts to improve the methodological and empirical basis for the measurement of population health, and has initiated a data collection strategy consisting of household and/or postal or telephone surveys in representative samples of the general populations using a standardized instrument together with new statistical methods for correcting biases in self-reported health (Ustun et al., 2001).

In constructing estimates of healthy life expectancy for 191 countries for the year 2000, we have sought to address some of the methodological challenges regarding comparability of health status data across populations and cultures. This paper briefly describes methods and data sources used to prepare the DALE estimates for the 191 member countries of WHO, and then examines the implications of the results for our understanding of global patterns of female-male differences in healthy life expectancy at age 60, and their proximate disease and injury causes.

METHODS

Calculation of healthy life expectancy requires three inputs. First, life expectancy at each age is calculated in the standard way. Second, estimates of the prevalence of various states of health at each age are required. Finally, a method of valuing this time compared to full health must be developed. Data and methods for each of these components is briefly described below. Because comparable health status prevalence data are not yet available for all countries, a three-stage strategy was used to estimate severity-weighted health state prevalences for countries:

- first, data from the Global Burden of Disease 2000 study (GBD2000) were used to estimate severity-adjusted disability prevalences by age and sex for all 191 countries;
- second, data on health state prevalences and health state valuations from the WHO survey program was used to make independent estimates of severity-adjusted disability prevalences by age and sex for 55 countries;
- finally, for the survey countries, "posterior" prevalences were calculated as weighted averages of the GBD2000-based prevalences and the survey prevalences. The relationship between the GBD 2000-based prevalences and the survey prevalence among the survey countries was then used to adjust the GBD2000-based prevalences for the non-survey countries.

Life Tables and Cause of Death Distributions for Countries

New life tables and detailed cause of death distributions were developed for all 191 WHO Member States for the year 2000, starting with a systematic review of all available evidence from surveys, censuses, sample registration systems, population laboratories, and national vital registration systems on levels and trends of child and adult mortality (Lopez et al., 2000). In countries with a substantial HIV epidemic, separate estimates were made of the numbers and distributions of deaths due to HIV/AIDS and these deaths incorporated into the life table estimates (Salomon et al., 2000). Causes of death for the 191 WHO member states were estimated based on data from national vital registration systems that capture about 17 million deaths annually. In addition, information from sample registration systems, population laboratories, and epidemiological analyses of specific conditions have been used to improve estimates of the cause of death patterns. Cause of death patterns were carefully analyzed to take into account incomplete coverage of vital registration in countries and the likely differences in cause of death patterns that would be expected in the low coverage areas of countries with incomplete data (Salomon & Murray, 2000).

GBD2000 Estimates of Severity-Weighted Disability for Countries

WHO is currently updating and revising estimates of the Global Burden of Disease for the year 2000. The burden of disease methodology provides a way to link information at the population level on disease causes and occurrence to information on both short-term and long-term health outcomes, including impairments, disability, and death (Murray & Lopez, 1996). These revisions draw on a wide range of data sources, and various methods have been developed to reconcile often fragmented and partial estimates of epidemiological parameters that are available from different studies (Mathers, Lopez et al., 2001). These data, together with the new and revised estimates of deaths by cause, age, and sex for all member states, were used to develop internally consistent estimates of incidence, prevalence, duration, and YLD (years lived with disability), for over 130 major causes, for 17 sub-regions of the 6 WHO regions of the world. As well as the usual incidence-based YLD, prevalence rates and prevalence-based YLD rates were also calculated by cause, age, and sex, giving direct estimates of the severity-weighted prevalence of health states attributable to each cause (Mathers, Murray et al., 2000). These estimates are used here to examine the patterns of causes of disability in older women in different regions of the world, and to contrast them with the causes of disability in older men.

The regional YLD rates from the Global Burden of Disease 2000 project were also used to estimate country-specific YLD rates by age and sex for the calculation of HALE. Where feasible, country-specific prevalence estimates were made for a number of causes (including childhood immunizable diseases, malnutrition, HIV/AIDS, cancers, and diabetes). For other causes, regional disability estimates were used, together with country-specific cause of death information, to develop country-specific estimates of severity-weighted prevalence of health states of less than good health (Mathers, Murray et al., 2000).

Summation of prevalence YLD over all causes would result in over-estimation of disability prevalence because of comorbidity between conditions. We corrected for independent comorbidity between major cause groups as follows:

$$D_{s,x} = 1 - \prod_g (1 - PYLD_{s,x,g})$$

where $PYLD_{s,x,g}$ is the prevalence YLD per 1000 population for sex s, age x and cause g and $D_{s,x}$ gives the overall severity-weighted prevalence of disability by age and sex.

Health Survey Data

In order to gather population health data in a truly comparable manner across all member states, WHO launched a survey study in 1999 through a series of carefully designed steps (Ustun et al., 2001). The health module was based on selected domains of the International Classification of Functioning, Disability, and Health (ICF). It was developed after a rigorous scientific review of various existing assessment instruments, international consultations with experts, and with representatives of national and international statistical agencies, and has been informed by the scientific literature and pilot studies in 10 countries.

Comparability is fundamental to the use of survey results for calculating summary measures of population health but has been underemphasized in instrument development. The WHO survey program has at its first objective the assessment of health in different domains for nationally representative adult population samples in a way that is comparable across populations. To do this, the survey includes case vignettes and some measured tests on selected domains that are intended to calibrate the description that respondents provide of their own health.

WHO has developed statistical methods for correcting biases in self-reported health using these data, based on the hierarchical ordered probit (HOPIT) model (Murray et al., 2000). The calibrated responses for 63 surveys in 55 countries were used to estimate the true prevalence of different states of health by age and sex for the HALE estimates reported here (Mathers, Murray et al., 2000).

Just over one half (34) of the surveys were household interview surveys, two were telephone surveys, and the remainder postal surveys. Thirty-five of the surveys were carried out in 31 European countries, 22 surveys in 19 developing countries, and the remainder in Canada, USA, Australia, and New Zealand.

Valuing Health States

A related objective of the WHO survey is to measure the value that individuals assign to descriptions of health states derived from decrements in major domains of body functions and activities. This allows the weighting of health states in calculating summary measures such as HALE. The WHO survey program uses a two-tiered data collection strategy involving the general population surveys described above, combined with more detailed surveys among respondents with high levels of educational attainment in the same sites.

In the household surveys, individuals provide descriptions for a series of hypothetical health states along seven core domains of health, listed in Table 1, followed by valuations of these states using a simple thermometer-type (visual analog) scale. The more detailed surveys include more abstract and cognitively demanding valuation tasks (standard gamble, time trade-off, and person trade-off) that have limited reliability in general population surveys but have been applied widely in industrialized countries among convenience samples of educated respondents.

TABLE 1. Core Domains of Health Used in WHO Health Status Survey Module for Measurement and Valuation of Health States

Health Domains	
1. Mobility	4. Pain and discomfort
2. Self-care	5. Affect (anxiety/depression)
3. Usual activities	6. Cognition

Statistical methods have been used to estimate the relationships between valuations elicited using visual analog scale and those elicited with other valuation techniques in order to measure the underlying health state severities that inform responses on each of the different measurement methods. A valuation function based on estimation of the relationships between levels on the core domains of health for a particular health state and the valuation of that health state has then been used together with the calibrated prevalences of health states to estimate the overall severity-weighted prevalence of health states for the 61 surveys in 55 countries (Mathers, Murray et al., 2000).

Posterior Health State Prevalences for the Calculation of HALE

The prevalence estimates for all 191 countries based on the GBD-based prior estimates (described above) and the prevalence estimates for the countries with health surveys were combined using Bayesian methods to obtain posterior health state prevalences for all Member States. Bayesian statistical analysis techniques use evidence (the health surveys) together with prior probability distributions (the GBD-based prevalence estimates) to calculate new posterior probability distributions. Both the evidence (survey mean severity-weighted prevalences by age and sex) and the prior means were assumed to be normally distributed, allowing the posterior mean severity-weighted prevalence to be calculated as the weighted sum of the survey mean and the prior mean, where the weights are inversely proportional to the standard errors of the uncertainties for each (Mathers, Murray et al., 2000).

Evidence from the surveys was also used to update the prior estimates for non-survey countries. Least squares ordinary regression was used to model the relationship between the posterior prevalences and the prior prevalences for the survey countries. The fitted model was then used to estimate posterior severity-weighted prevalences for all non-survey countries, in order to (1) ensure that the use of the survey data did not introduce a prevalence differential between survey and non-survey countries, and (2) to take the survey evidence into account in making the best possible prevalence estimates for non-survey countries.

Calculation of HALE

HALE was calculated using Sullivan's method based on abridged country life tables and the posterior estimates of severity-weighted prevalence of disability (Mathers, Murray et al., 2000). Uncertainty distributions for the HALE estimates for each country were also calculated to take into account uncertainty in the life table quantities and in the posterior prevalence estimates (Salomon et al., 2001).

RESULTS

Japanese older women lead the world with an estimated average healthy life expectancy of 21.4 years at age 60 in 2000 (Table 2). HALE for Japanese males aged 60 years is 3.8 years lower at 17.6 years. This a narrower gap than for total life expectancy at age 65 years of 5.4 years. After Japan, in second to fifth places, are Monaco, San Marino, Switzerland, Australia, and France with healthy life expectancies of older women in the range 19.4 to 20.2 years, followed by a number of other industrialized countries of Western Europe. Full details of male and female HALE and total life expectancy at age 60, together with 95% uncertainty ranges, are available by country in the World Health Report 2001 (WHO 2001).

Overall, global healthy life expectancy for women at age 60 in 2000 is 14.1 years, just over 2 years greater than that for men (Table 3). In comparison, total life expectancy at age 60 is 20.2 years, almost 4 years higher than that for men. HALE at age 60 ranges from a low of 6.3 years for African women to a high of just over 24 years in the low mortality countries of mainly Western Europe and North America. This is a 4-fold difference in healthy life expectancy between major regional populations of the world. The difference between HALE and total life expectancy is HLE (healthy life expectancy "lost" due to disability). HLE for women aged 60 ranges from 47% (of total life expectancy at birth) in Africa to 22% in the European region.

Apart from Afghanistan (where female healthy life expectancy at age 60 is just 5.8 years), the bottom 10 countries are all in sub-Saharan Africa, where the HIV-AIDS epidemic is rampant and there is a high disability burden due to chronic diseases and injury, as well as to other communicable diseases and childhood and maternal causes earlier in life.

Figure 1 shows HALE at birth for women versus men for the 191 countries in the year 2000. In the countries with HALE at birth of 46 years or lower, male and female HALE are almost the same. These countries are almost entirely African countries, but include the Lao People's Republic, Haiti, and Nepal. There are a number of countries with

TABLE 2. Healthy Life Expectancy for Women Aged 60 years, WHO Member States, 2000

Rank	Member State	HALE (years)	Rank	Member State	HALE (years)	Rank	Member State	HALE (years)
1	Japan	21.4	65	Cyprus	14.1	129	Nauru	10.5
2	Monaco	20.2	66	Saint Vincent and Grenadines	14.1	130	Papua New Guinea	10.5
3	San Marino	19.9	67	Slovakia	14.0	131	South Africa	10.4
4	Switzerland	19.7	68	Paraguay	14.0	132	Tajikistan	10.3
5	Australia	19.5	69	Colombia	14.0	133	Cambodia	10.1
6	France	19.4	70	Saint Lucia	13.9	134	Egypt	10.0
7	Andorra	19.3	71	Hungary	13.8	135	Morocco	10.0
8	Sweden	18.9	72	Niue	13.8	136	Bolivia	10.0
9	Italy	18.8	73	Poland	13.8	137	Myanmar	9.8
10	New Zealand	18.6	74	Belize	13.6	138	Zimbabwe	9.7
11	Iceland	18.6	75	Tonga	13.6	139	Swaziland	9.6
12	Austria	18.4	76	Philippines	13.6	140	Nepal	9.6
13	Luxembourg	18.4	77	Peru	13.6	141	Iraq	9.6
14	Spain	18.3	78	Turkey	13.4	142	Turkmenistan	9.5
15	Norway	18.2	79	Trinidad and Tobago	13.3	143	Gabon	9.3
16	Belgium	18.0	80	United Arab Emirates	13.3	144	Sao Tome and Principe	9.2
17	Finland	17.9	81	Suriname	13.3	145	Namibia	9.1
18	Netherlands	17.8	82	El Salvador	13.3	146	Kenya	9.1
19	Canada	17.8	83	Cook Islands	13.0	147	Ghana	9.0
20	Malta	17.7	84	Dominican Republic	13.0	148	Botswana	8.9
21	Greece	17.6	85	Kuwait	13.0	149	Congo	8.9
22	Germany	17.6	86	Mongolia	12.7	150	Lesotho	8.8
23	United Kingdom	17.4	87	Malaysia	12.7	151	Yemen	8.8
24	Israel	17.1	88	Honduras	12.7	152	Pakistan	8.7
25	USA	16.9	89	Fiji	12.7	153	Maldives	8.6
26	Ireland	16.9	90	Tunisia	12.6	154	Togo	8.6
27	Slovenia	16.7	91	Saint Kitts and Nevis	12.6	155	Haiti	8.5
28	Denmark	16.5	92	Bahamas	12.6	156	Bhutan	8.5
29	Dominica	16.4	93	Brazil	12.6	157	Cote d'Ivoire	8.5
30	Singapore	16.2	94	Nicaragua	12.5	158	Zambia	8.5
31	Barbados	16.1	95	Republic of Moldova	12.5	159	Equatorial Guinea	8.3
32	Portugal	16.0	96	Indonesia	12.5	160	Nigeria	8.2

Rank	Country	Value	Rank	Country	Value	Rank	Country	Value
33	Argentina	16.0	97	Solomon Islands	12.4	161	Eritrea	8.1
34	Republic of Korea	16.0	98	Viet Nam	12.3	162	Gambia	8.1
35	Costa Rica	15.9	99	Marshall Islands	12.3	163	Bangladesh	8.0
36	Uruguay	15.8	100	Mauritius	12.3	164	Cameroon	8.0
37	Czech Republic	15.8	101	Russian Federation	12.2	165	Senegal	8.0
38	Chile	15.7	102	Lebanon	12.2	166	Central African Republic	7.9
39	Jamaica	15.7	103	Saudi Arabia	12.1	167	Malawi	7.8
40	Cuba	15.5	104	DPR Korea (b)	12.1	168	Sudan	7.8
41	Antigua and Barbuda	15.4	105	Oman	12.1	169	Comoros	7.7
42	Panama	15.3	106	Armenia	12.0	170	Burundi	7.7
43	Bulgaria	15.2	107	Micronesia (Fed. States of)	12.0	171	United Rep. of Tanzania	7.7
44	Croatia	15.2	108	Cape Verde	12.0	172	Ethiopia	7.5
45	Mexico	15.1	109	Ukraine	11.8	173	Madagascar	7.5
46	Brunei Darussalam	15.1	110	Kyrgyzstan	11.8	174	Chad	7.5
47	Estonia	14.8	111	Bahrain	11.8	175	Uganda	7.4
48	Venezuela	14.7	112	Guatemala	11.7	176	Burkina Faso	7.4
49	Sri Lanka	14.6	113	Vanuatu	11.7	177	Benin	7.4
50	Azerbaijan	14.6	114	Uzbekistan	11.6	178	Dem. Republic of the Congo	7.4
51	Kazakhstan	14.6	115	Qatar	11.6	179	Mozambique	7.3
52	Yugoslavia	14.6	116	Tuvalu	11.5	180	Angola	7.3
53	Albania	14.4	117	Iran (Islamic Republic of)	11.4	181	Rwanda	7.2
54	Latvia	14.4	118	Kiribati	11.4	182	Mali	7.2
55	Ecuador	14.4	119	Syrian Arab Republic	11.3	183	Guinea-Bissau	7.1
56	Belarus	14.4	120	Libyan Arab Jamahiriya	11.3	184	Mauritania	7.1
57	Thailand	14.4	121	Jordan	11.3	185	Guinea	7.0
58	Romania	14.4	122	Guyana	11.1	186	Djibouti	7.0
59	China	14.3	123	Georgia	11.1	187	Liberia	6.9
60	Samoa	14.3	124	Algeria	11.0	188	Somalia	6.4
61	Bosnia and Herzegovina	14.3	125	India	10.9	189	Sierra Leone	6.0
62	TFYR Macedonia (a)	14.3	126	Seychelles	10.7	190	Afghanistan	5.8
63	Lithuania	14.2	127	Palau	10.7	191	Niger	5.8
64	Grenada	14.1	128	Lao People's Dem. Republic	10.6			

(a) The Former Yugoslav Republic of Macedonia (b) Democratic People's Republic of Korea

TABLE 3. Life Expectancy (LE), Healthy Life Expectancy (HALE), and Lost Healthy Years as Percent of Total LE (LHE%), at Birth and at Age 60, by Sex and Region, 2000

Region[a]	Females			Males			Female-Male Difference		
	HALE (years)	LE (years)	LHE% (%)	HALE (years)	LE (years)	LHE% (%)	HALE (years)	LE (years)	LHE% (%)
At birth									
Low mortality countries	72.0	81.2	11.4	68.0	75.1	9.5	4.0	6.1	1.9
Eastern Europe	61.0	72.2	15.5	54.0	62.9	14.2	7.0	9.3	1.3
Latin America	61.8	73.7	16.1	58.0	67.0	13.4	3.8	6.7	2.7
Eastern Mediterranean	55.9	69.4	19.5	56.4	66.1	14.7	−0.6	3.3	4.8
Asia/Pacific	57.5	67.6	15.0	56.2	63.9	12.2	1.3	3.6	2.8
Africa	38.9	48.8	20.3	39.5	47.0	15.9	−0.6	1.9	4.4
World	57.0	67.2	15.1	54.9	62.7	12.5	2.1	4.5	2.7
At age 60									
Low mortality countries	18.8	24.2	22.4	15.9	19.9	19.8	2.9	4.4	2.6
Eastern Europe	13.0	18.9	31.5	9.6	14.6	34.2	3.3	4.3	−2.7
Latin America	14.1	20.8	32.2	12.3	17.5	29.9	1.8	3.3	2.2
Eastern Mediterranean	10.3	18.0	42.4	10.4	16.1	35.5	0.0	1.9	6.9
Asia/Pacific	12.9	19.0	32.2	11.1	15.9	29.8	1.7	3.1	2.4
Africa	8.3	15.8	47.3	8.3	13.9	40.2	0.0	1.9	7.1
World	14.1	20.2	30.3	11.9	16.7	28.3	2.2	3.6	2.0

[a]*Low mortality countries* include Western Europe, North America, Japan, Australia, New Zealand, Singapore, and Brunei Darussalam; *Eastern Europe* includes Turkey and the former socialist countries of Eastern Europe and Central Asia; *Asia/Pacific* includes India, China, and other Asian and Pacific countries apart from the four included in *Low mortality countries*; *Africa* includes the countries of sub-Saharan Africa; North African countries are included in *Eastern Mediterranean*.

HALE around 50 years, where female HALE at birth is actually lower than male HALE. These countries are mostly in North Africa or the Eastern Mediterranean region, but also include Afghanistan, Pakistan, and Bangladesh. For other countries with HALE at birth of greater than 50 years, female HALE is generally higher than male HALE, though the gap is lower than for total life expectancy. In many countries of Eastern Europe, female HALE at birth is substantially higher than male, reflecting very high levels of adult mortality in men in the 1990s.

In Russia in the year 2000, healthy life expectancy is estimated to be 60.6 years for females, 4 years below the European average, but just 50.3 years for males, 9 years below the European average. This is one of the widest sex gaps in the world and reflects the sharp increase in adult male mortality in the early 1990s. Similar rates exist for other countries of the former Soviet Union.

FIGURE 1. Healthy Life Expectancy at Birth for Females versus Males, 191 Countries, 2000

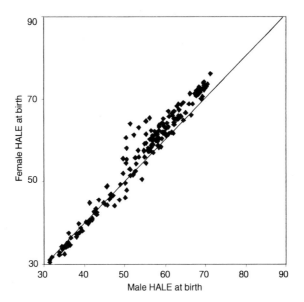

Similar patterns are apparent for the male-female gap in healthy life expectancy at age 60 (Figure 2), although the male-female reversal in Eastern Mediterranean countries no longer occurs. In the countries with the longest healthy life expectancies, there is a trend to increasing female-male gap with increasing HALE, reflecting the greater proportion of years of life lived at older ages by women aged 60 and over, where there are higher prevalences of disabling conditions such as dementia and musculoskeletal disorders.

As shown in Figure 3, the gap between female HALE at age 60 and total life expectancy at age 60 decreases with increasing life expectancy in the developing countries, reflecting declining prevalence of disability due to communicable, maternal, perinatal, and nutritional causes. Among countries with higher life expectancies, the gap stabilizes and there is some indication that it may start to widen in the countries with the highest life expectancies. This may reflect the increasing burden of

FIGURE 2. Healthy Life Expectancy (HALE) at Age 60 for Females versus Males, 191 Countries, 2000

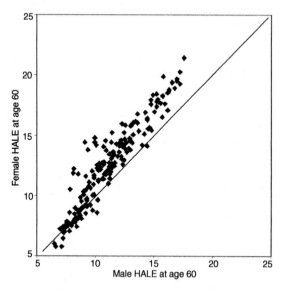

FIGURE 3. Healthy Life Expectancy (HALE) at Age 60 versus Total Life Expectancy at Age 60, Females, 191 Countries, 2000

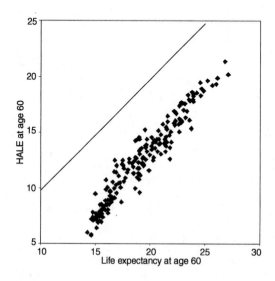

disability at older ages from non-fatal conditions such as musculoskeletal disorders, neuropsychiatric conditions, and sense organ disorders, as well as the increasing disability associated with the major causes of mortality (cardiovascular diseases and respiratory diseases in particular).

Figure 4 summarize the changing patterns of causes of disability in older females across the world, as assessed by the Global Burden of Disease 2000 project. The figure shows the major causes of prevalence YLD per 1000 population for 6 groups of countries. Prevalence YLD measure the equivalent healthy years of life lost due to disability resulting from diseases and injuries. Group 1 conditions (communicable, maternal, perinatal, and nutritional causes) are an important cause of disability for older women in Africa and the Middle East. Among the low mortality populations of Eastern and Western Europe, North America, Japan, Australia, and New Zealand, neuropsychiatric conditions and other non-communicable diseases are the dominant causes of disability at older ages.

Table 4 shows the top 15 disease and injury causes of disability (prevalence YLD) for older women in developed countries (the low mortality countries plus Eastern Europe) and in developing countries (the rest of the world). In developed countries, senile dementias are responsible for over 20% of loss of healthy life, and YLD rates are 40% higher for females than males. Osteoarthritis is the second leading cause

FIGURE 4. YLD per 1,000 Population by Major Cause Group, Females Aged 60 Years and Over, by Region, 2000. Group 1 Conditions Include Communicable, Maternal, Perinatal, and Nutritional Conditions

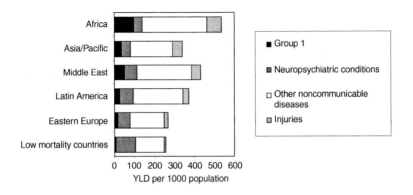

TABLE 4. Top 15 Causes of Disability (YLD), for Women Aged 60 Years and Over, Developed and Developing Countries,[a] 2000

	% of total YLD	Female to male ratio[b]
Developed countries		
1 Alzheimer and other dementias*	21.3	1.41
2 Osteoarthritis	11.2	1.47
3 Hearing loss, adult onset	7.0	0.86
4 Cerebrovascular disease	5.8	1.15
5 Unipolar depressive disorders	3.6	1.80
6 Diabetes mellitus	3.4	1.07
7 Chronic obstructive pulmonary disease	2.9	0.44
8 Malignant neoplasms	2.3	0.58
9 Ischaemic heart disease	1.9	0.77
10 Falls	1.6	0.64
11 Maternal conditions	1.4	---
12 Parkinson's disease	1.5	0.88
13 Oral conditions	1.4	1.49
14 Migraine	1.4	2.42
15 Rheumatoid arthritis	1.3	2.15
Developing countries		
1 Chronic obstructive pulmonary disease	9.9	0.74
2 Cataracts	7.3	1.11
3 Osteoarthritis	7.2	1.36
4 Hearing loss, adult onset	7.0	0.75
5 Alzheimer and other dementias	4.7	1.03
6 Falls	3.2	0.75
7 Unipolar depressive disorders	2.9	1.79
8 Maternal conditions	2.8	---
9 Cerebrovascular disease	2.7	1.23
10 Ischaemic heart disease	2.2	1.06
11 Perinatal conditions*	2.2	0.94
12 Oral conditions	1.9	1.09
13 Diabetes mellitus	1.7	0.89
14 Iron-deficiency anàemia	1.5	0.99
15 Road traffic accidents	1.5	0.34

[a] Developed countries include European countries, Canada, USA, Japan, Australia, New Zealand.
[b] Ratio of total YLD per 1,000 population for females aged 60 years and over to those for males aged 60 years and over.

of YLD, again with a female excess compared to males, followed by hearing loss, where the female rate is 14% lower than the male rate.

In developing countries, in contrast, chronic obstructive lung disease is the leading cause of disability burden in older women, responsible for around 10% of the total. This reflects the impact of both smoking and indoor air pollution. Cataracts are the second leading cause, reflecting the high burden of blindness in the developing world due to unoperated cataracts in older people. Perinatal and maternal conditions also cause significant disability in older women, unlike in developed countries.

DISCUSSION

Despite the fact that women live longer in the richer, more developed countries, and have greater opportunity to acquire non-fatal disabilities in older age, disability has a greater absolute (and relative) impact on healthy life expectancy at age 60 in poorer countries. Separating life expectancy into equivalent years of good health and years of lost good health thus widens rather than narrows the difference in health status between the rich and the poor countries. Cross-sectionally, at the global level, higher life expectancy at age 60 is associated with a compression of morbidity in developing countries: fewer expected years of good health are lost due to the non-fatal consequences of diseases and injury as mortality rates decline. There is some indication in these data that there may be some expansion of morbidity cross-sectionally with increasing life expectancy at older ages in the low mortality countries.

At a global level, older women live on average 3.6 years longer than men, but lose the equivalent of 1.4 extra years of good health to the non-fatal consequences of diseases and injuries. In other words, although females live longer, they spend a greater amount of time with disability. However, this global average disguises enormous variations across the world in the sex difference in healthy life expectancy. The male-female gap in healthy life expectancy at age 60 varies from a high of 10 years in some former Soviet Union countries to a low of −1.5 years for some Middle Eastern countries.

Russia has one of the widest sex gaps in the world for healthy life expectancy of older people: 66.4 years for females at birth but just 56.1 years for males. The most common explanation is the high incidence of male alcohol abuse, which led to high rates of accidents, violence, and cardiovascular disease. From 1987 to 1994, the risk of premature death increased by 70% for Russian males. Between 1994 and 1998, life expectancy improved for males, but has gotten worse in the last few years.

In some countries of North Africa, the Middle East, and West Asia, the gap in healthy life expectancy at birth for males and females is reversed. Contributing to these sex differences are higher female infant and child mortality rates, and higher risks of maternal mortality than in other countries, reflecting the position of women in these societies.

As with any innovative approach, there are substantial limitations and gaps in the information base required for estimating healthy life expectancy for all countries of the world. We have attempted to maximize the comparability of the data derived from available, nationally representative health surveys, and have used additional cross-population comparable information on health status derived from analysis of epidemiological data sources to improve comparability.

The WHO instrument has been used to collect population health data in over 50 countries at the time of writing, and this experience will be used to improve the health status measurement methods and to extend the surveys to more countries. In addition, WHO is investing considerable resources in the revision of the Global Burden of Disease estimates for the year 2000. These estimates will also contribute to improved estimation of healthy life expectancy, which will in turn assist in monitoring global health trends, and in particular, trends in the health and healthy life expectancy of older women.

REFERENCES

Lopez, A. D., Salomon, J., Ahmad, O., & Murray, C. J. L. (2000). *Life tables for 191 countries: Data, methods and results.* GPE discussion Paper No. 9. Geneva: World Health Organization; 2000. Also available on the worldwide web at *www.who.int/evidence.*

Mathers, C. D., Lopez, A. D., Murray, C. J. L., & Stein, C. (2001). *The Global Burden of Disease 2000 project: Aims, methods and data sources.* GPE Discussion Paper No. 36. Geneva: World Health Organization. Also available on the worldwide web at *www.who.int/evidence.*

Mathers, C. D., Murray, C. J. L., Salomon, J., & Lopez, A. D. (2001). *Estimates of healthy life expectancy for 191 countries in the year 2000: Methods and results.* GPE Discussion Paper No. 38. Geneva: World Health Organization. Also available on the worldwide web at *www.who.int/evidence.*

Mathers, C. D., Sadana, R., Salomon, J., Murray, C. J. L., & Lopez, A. D. (2001). *Healthy life expectancy in 191 countries, 1999.* The Lancet 357: 1685-1691.

Murray, C. J. L., & Lopez, A. D. (Ed.). (1996). *The global burden of disease: A comprehensive assessment of mortality and disability from diseases, injuries and risk factors in 1990 and projected to 2020.* Global Burden of Disease and Injury Series, Vol. 1. Cambridge: Harvard University Press; 1996.

Murray, C. J. L., Tandon, A., Salomon, J., & Mathers, C. D. (2000). *Enhancing cross-population comparability of survey results.* GPE Discussion Paper No. 35. Geneva: World Health Organization. Also available on the worldwide web at *www.who.int/evidence.*

Murray, C. J. L., Salomon, J., Mathers, C. D., & Lopez, A. D. (Ed.) (2001). *Summary measures of population health.* Geneva: World Health Organization 2001.

Robine, J.M., Mathers, C. D., & Brouard, N. (1996). *Trends and differentials in disability-free life expectancy: Concepts, methods and findings.* In Caselli G., Lopez A. (Ed.). Health and Mortality Among Elderly Populations (pp. 182-201). Oxford: Clarendon Press.

Sadana, R., Mathers, C. D., Lopez, A. D., Murray, C. J. L., & Iberg, K. (2000). *Comparative analysis of more than 50 household surveys on health status.* GPE discussion Paper No. 15. Geneva: World Health Organization. Also available on the worldwide web at *www.who.int/evidence.*

Salomon, J., Gakidou, E. E., & Murray, C. J. L. (2000). *Methods for modelling the HIV/AIDS epidemic in sub-Saharan Africa.* GPE discussion Paper No. 3. Geneva: World Health Organization. Also available on the worldwide web at *www.who.int/evidence.*

Salomon, J. & Murray, C. J. L. (2000). *Compositional models for mortality by age, sex and cause.* GPE discussion Paper No. 11. Geneva: World Health Organization. Also available on the worldwide web at *www.who.int/evidence.*

Salomon, J. S., Mathers, C. D., Murray, C. J. L., & Ferguson, B. (2001). *Methods for life expectancy and healthy life expectancy uncertainty analysis.* GPE discussion paper No. 10. Geneva, World Health Organization. Also available on the worldwide web at *www.who.int/evidence.*

Üstün, T. B., Chatterji, S., Villanueva, M., Bendib, L., Celik, C., Sadana, R., Valentine, N., Mathers, C., Ortiz, J., Tandon, A., Salomon, J., Yang, C., Xie Wan, J., & Murray, C. J. L. (2001). *WHO Multi-Country Household Survey Study on Health and Responsiveness, 2000-2001.* GPE discussion paper No. 37. Geneva, World Health Organization. Also available on the worldwide web at *www. who.int/evidence.*

World Health Organization. (2000). *World Health Report 2000. Health systems: Improving performance.* Geneva: World Health Organization. Also available on the worldwide web at *www.who.int/whr.*

World Health Organization. (2001). *World Health Report 2001. Mental health: New understanding, new hope.* Geneva, World Health Organization. Also available on the worldwide web at *www.who.int/whr.*

European Perspectives
on Healthy Aging in Women

Jean-Marie Robine, DED
Carol Jagger, PhD
Emmanuelle Cambois, PhD

SUMMARY. Using data from the 1994 European Community Household Panel, we compare active life expectancy differentials at age 65 years between women and men in 12 European countries. We seek to explain the extent to which differences are a reflection of gender differentials in life expectancy at 65 years or reflect differences in active life expectancy earlier in life. Considerable variation in the gender differentials in both total and active life expectancies at age 65 years exist within Europe, with some countries experiencing 20% lower life expectancy at age 65 years for men compared to women. Some evidence was found to suggest that gender differentials in active life expectancy may continue from younger ages through to later life. *[Article copies available for a fee from The Haworth Document Delivery Service: 1-800-HAWORTH. E-mail address: <getinfo@haworthpressinc.com> Website: <http://www.HaworthPress. com> © 2002 by The Haworth Press, Inc. All rights reserved.]*

Jean-Marie Robine and Emmanuelle Cambois are affiliated with the Health and Demography team in the Department of Biostatistics, University of Montpellier I, France.

Carol Jagger is Professor of Epidemiology in the Department of Epidemiology and Public Health at the University of Leicester, England.

Address correspondence to: Jean-Marie Robine, Senior Research Fellow, INSERM Démographie et Santé, Val d'Aurelle, Parc Euromédecine, 34298 Montpellier Cedex 5, France (E-mail: robine@valdorel.fnclcc.fr).

[Haworth co-indexing entry note]: "European Perspectives on Healthy Aging in Women." Robine, Jean-Marie, Carol Jagger, and Emmanuelle Cambois. Co-published simultaneously in *Journal of Women & Aging* (The Haworth Press, Inc.) Vol. 14, No. 1/2, 2002, pp. 119-133; and: *Health Expectations for Older Women: International Perspectives* (ed: Sarah B. Laditka) The Haworth Press, Inc., 2002, pp. 119-133. Single or multiple copies of this article are available for a fee from The Haworth Document Delivery Service [1-800-HAWORTH 9:00 a.m. - 5:00 p.m. (EST). E-mail address: getinfo@haworthpressinc.com].

119

KEYWORDS. Active life expectancy, disability-free life expectancy, mortality, life expectancy, European Community Household Panel

INTRODUCTION

Health expectancies are now increasingly used in industrialized countries to assess the evolution of the populations' health status, in particular that of older people and estimates of health expectancy (generally, disability-free life expectancy) are available for 49 countries (Robine, Romieu, and Cambois, 1999), including many European Union Member States. Gender differentials in life expectancy and disability-free life expectancy within Europe have been noted but not examined themselves in depth, most research has been within European countries and has focused on regional, time, or socio-economic differences in health expectancies (Perenboom, Boshuizen, and van de Water, 1993; Bone et al., 1995; Van Oyen, Tafforeau, and Roelands, 1996; Sihvonen et al., 1998; Bronnum-Hansen, 2000; Melzer et al., 2000). In general, gender differences in life expectancy are greater than with disability-free life expectancy with women living longer in total and without disability, although as a proportion of their total remaining life expectancy women tend to spend a shorter time without disability compared to men (van Ginneken, Dissevelt, van de Water, and van Sonsbeek, 1991; Romieu and Robine, 1994).

Many of these estimates are not directly comparable however, even within countries over time, since there is a large variation in the definitions of disability used in different national surveys, in addition to differences in survey design. Survey factors that may impact on the prevalence of disability found in different surveys includes mode of interview (self-report, interviewer, or telephone), response rate, level of proxy respondents, and whether or not institutionalized older people are included.

Within the European Union (EU), the introduction of the European Community Household Panel (ECHP) has enhanced the collection of comparable data across the EU Member States. This longitudinal, multi-subject survey covers many aspects of daily life, including employment, income, education, and health, and was designed to complement the two main surveys at EU level: the labour force survey and the household income survey. Several health questions are included in the ECHP, including a general question on restrictions in activities of daily living (Verbrugge, 1997).

The aim of this study is, therefore, to compare the gender differentials in active life expectancy across the European countries using the same survey design and question to overcome previous problems of comparability. We also examine the extent to which any differences in active life expectancy between men and women at earlier ages contribute to any gender differences found at age 65 years. Geographical patterns in the relationship between life expectancy and active life expectancy are investigated since notable differences between the Nordic and southern European countries exist in diet, for instance, the benefits of the Mediterranean diet (Trichopoulou and Vasilopoulou, 2000), as well as differences in education, health behaviours, and attitudes to health (Kafatos et al., 1999).

METHODS

Two sets of data are required to calculate active life expectancy: the age- and sex-specific prevalence of activity restriction and period life tables. The data on activity restriction are taken from the first wave, in 1994, of the ECHP, covering twelve Member States of the European Union at the time the survey was planned: Belgium, Denmark, Eire (the Republic of Ireland), France, Germany, Greece, Italy, Luxembourg, The Netherlands, Portugal, Spain, and the United Kingdom. The reference wording in English for the question used to assess activity restriction is: "Are you hampered in your daily activities by any chronic physical or mental health problem, illness, or disability?" with responses "Yes, severely," "Yes, to some extent," "No." Further details of the ECHP can be found in Eurostat (1996). National mortality data was supplied by Eurostat and relate to 1994.

Active life expectancies were calculated using Sullivan's method (Sullivan, 1971). However, since the ECHP interviews only adults aged 16 years and over in households, two assumptions have been made. First, because of the lack of comparable data on institutional residents in the Member States, we have assumed that years lived in an institution are partitioned into years lived with and without disability in the same proportions as those living in the community (Robine and Mormiche, 1994). Second, in order to present estimates at birth, we have, in all counties, applied a constant disability rate of 1% between the ages of 0 and 16. This rate, compatible with the values observed over the age of 16 years, has virtually no impact on the value of active life expectancy.

We wished to explore whether gender differences in active life expectancies at age 65 were associated with gender differences in active and total life expectancies at birth. However, the values at birth are obviously correlated with the values at age 65 years as the latter form a part of the values at birth. Thus, instead of the life expectancies and active life expectancies at birth, we used the temporal life expectancies and active life expectancies at birth, these being the values between birth and age 65 years. To then compare these values for men and women, we calculated the gender differences (female-male) as a percentage of female values for life expectancy, fully active life expectancy (defined as not restricted at all) and partly active life expectancy (defined as not severely restricted), all between birth and 65 years and at age 65 years. These quantities will be termed the "gender gap percentages." Percentages of female values were used rather than the gender differences themselves as the percentages were less correlated with the female values. For example, gender differences in life expectancy at age 65 were significantly correlated with female life expectancy at age 65 whilst the gender difference as a percentage of female life expectancy was not. We used Pearson correlation coefficients and linear regression to examine relationships between these quantities and to highlight patterns between countries.

We explored potential geographical patterns in the relationships between gender differentials in life expectancy and active life expectancy by relating these to the latitude of the capital city for each country. This would have the effect of highlighting any differences between the Nordic and Mediterranean countries if they exist.

RESULTS

Values of life expectancy (LE), fully active life expectancy (FALE) and partly active life expectancy (PALE) at age 65 for men and women are shown in Table 1. Rankings between countries are similar for men and women for LE and FALE but less so for PALE (free of severe restriction). Women in each country exceeded men on all life expectancies at age 65 years. Gender differences (female-male) in LE at 65 years ranged from 2.31 years (Greece) to 4.47 years (France). Active life expectancy differentials by gender at age 65 were greatest for PALE, which ranged from 1.77 years (Greece) to 3.85 years (Luxembourg), whilst FALE differences between women and men were almost zero (0.03 years) in Italy up to 1.55 years in Eire.

TABLE 1. Gender Differentials in Life Expectancy (LE),[1] Fully Active Life Expectancy,[1] and Partly Active Life Expectancy[2] at Age 65 Years, by Country

	LE at 65 years (rank)		Fully Active LE at 65 (rank)		Partly Active LE at 65 (rank)	
	Female	Male	Female	Male	Female	Male
Belgium	19.02 (4)	14.77 (5)	9.15 (6)	8.12 (8)	15.26 (4)	12.44 (5)
Denmark	17.71 (11)	14.26 (11)	9.17 (5)	8.86 (3)	14.77 (7)	12.40 (6)
Eire	17.32 (12)	13.82 (12)	9.81 (3)	8.26 (7)	15.80 (2)	12.36 (7)
France	20.61 (1)	16.13 (1)	10.30 (2)	8.84 (4)	14.72 (9)	11.86 (10)
Germany	18.32 (8)	14.63 (8)	7.87 (10)	6.50 (12)	14.42 (10)	11.44 (11)
Greece	18.37 (7)	16.06 (2)	9.67 (4)	8.66 (5)	14.77 (7)	13.00 (3)
Italy	19.21 (3)	15.43 (4)	7.62 (12)	7.59 (10)	14.23 (11)	12.16 (9)
Luxembourg	18.82 (6)	14.56 (9)	10.43 (1)	9.45 (1)	17.11 (1)	13.26 (2)
Netherlands	18.98 (5)	14.74 (6)	8.58 (8)	8.37 (6)	15.04 (5)	12.29 (8)
Portugal	17.76 (10)	14.40 (10)	7.88 (11)	7.15 (11)	13.93 (12)	11.43 (12)
Spain	19.74 (2)	15.95 (3)	9.06 (7)	8.96 (2)	15.43 (3)	13.63 (1)
United Kingdom	18.29 (9)	14.64 (7)	8.54 (9)	7.62 (9)	14.91 (6)	12.42 (4)

[1]Fully active life expectancy defined as life expectancy with no restrictions in activities
[2]Partly active life expectancy defined as life expectancy with no severe restrictions in activities

123

Gender gap percentages were much higher at age 65 than at earlier ages (Figure 1a) with the gender gap percentage in LE at age 65 being over 20% for seven of the twelve countries. When the gender gap percentages in LE, FALE, and PALE at age 65 years were looked at in relation to gender differentials at earlier ages, between birth and age 65 years, no consistent pattern was found either overall or by geographical area (Figure 1a), although there was some evidence that gender differentials in FALE and PALE at age 65 were smaller in the southern European countries (Spain, Portugal, Italy, Greece). It is interesting to note that the gender gap percentage in FALE between birth and age 65 was negative for four countries: Belgium, Denmark, Italy, and The Netherlands, showing that in these countries fully active life expectancy between birth and age 65 for men exceeded that for women.

To investigate the relationship between the gender differentials in FALE at age 65 years and values earlier in life, the gender gap percentages in LE and FALE between birth and age 65 and LE at age 65 were entered into a regression model with the gender gap percentage in FALE at age 65 as the dependent variable. The only significant association was with FALE between birth and age 65 (partial $r = 0.66$, $t = 2.48$, $p = 0.038$) with LE between birth and age 65 (partial $r = -0.22$, $t = -0.63$, $p = 0.55$) and LE at 65 (partial $r = 0.12$, $t = 0.33$, $p = 0.75$) showing little association with the gender gap percentage in FALE at age 65. These three variables accounted for 45% of the variation in the gender gap percentage in FALE at age 65. Gender differences in fully active life expectancy at age 65 seem thus to reflect the gender difference in fully active life expectancy at earlier ages. The association between FALE at age 65 and at earlier ages is shown in Figure 1b by country. In Denmark, The Netherlands, and Italy, the differences in FALE at age 65 between men and women were the least, and these countries also exhibited small differences between the sexes at earlier ages. In contrast, France, Germany, and Eire (the Republic of Ireland) had the largest gender differences in FALE at age 65 years and they also had the largest differences at younger ages.

Similar analyses were performed for gender gap percentage in partly active life expectancy (PALE) (defined as restricted not at all or to some extent) at age 65. For PALE, the only significant association was with LE at age 65 (partial $r = 0.65$, $t = 2.41$, $p = 0.04$), with little association with PALE between birth and age 65 (partial $r = 0.10$, $t = 0.28$, $p = 0.79$) or with LE between birth and age 65 (partial $r = -0.08$, $t = -0.21$, $p = 0.84$). These three variables accounted for 45% of the variation in the gender gap percentage in PALE at age 65. The bivariate association be-

FIGURE 1a. Gender Differentials in Life Expectancy (LE) Between Birth and Age 65 Years and at Age 65 Years, Alphabetically by Country

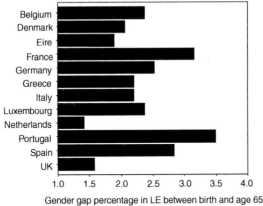

Gender gap percentage in LE between birth and age 65

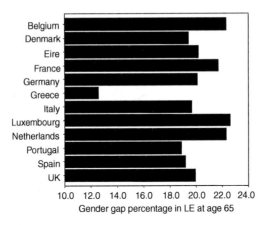

Gender gap percentage in LE at age 65

tween the gender gap percentage in PALE at age 65 and LE at age 65 is shown in Figure 1c. Noticeable in Figure 1c is the consistent position of Greece as having the second lowest gender gap percentages in PALE at age 65 (second to Spain), but also having the lowest gender gap percentage in LE at age 65. Indeed, this point had the highest leverage in the regression model and when omitted, there was no longer a significant association between the gender gap percentage in PALE at 65 and the gender gap percentage in LE at age 65.

FIGURE 1b. Gender Differentials in Fully Active Life Expectancy (FALE) Between Birth and Age 65 Years and at Age 65 Years, Alphabetically by Country

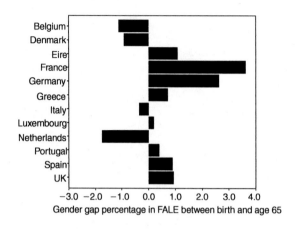

Gender gap percentage in FALE between birth and age 65

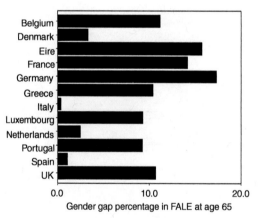

Gender gap percentage in FALE at age 65

The effect of geographical patterns, particularly north-south gradients on the gender gap percentages was investigated by looking at the relationship between these quantities and the latitude of the capital city for each country. No significant relationship was found for any of the gender gap percentages and latitude, suggesting no strong gradient north to south.

FIGURE 1c. Gender Differentials in Partly Active Life Expectancy (PALE) Between Birth and Age 65 and at Age 65 Years, Alphabetically by Country

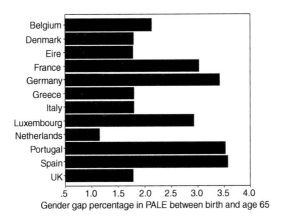

Gender gap percentage in PALE between birth and age 65

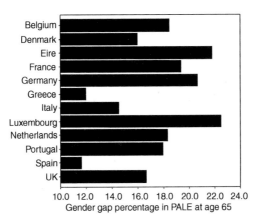

Gender gap percentage in PALE at age 65

DISCUSSION

Considerable differences between men and women in life expectancy and disability-free life expectancy at older ages were found within Europe. In some countries, the life expectancy of men aged 65 years was over 20% lower than that of women. In other studies, gender differences in disability-free life expectancy were generally smaller than those in life expectancy (Romieu and Robine, 1994). However, the correlations between life expectancy, fully active life expectancy, and partly active life expectancy at age 65 years were low, suggesting that a country that had small gender differences in life expectancy at age 65 did not necessarily also have small gender differences in active life expectancy (Figure 2). Although in general women's life expectancy and active life expectancy exceeded that of men, in four countries (Belgium, Denmark, Italy, and The Netherlands) this was not the case and the gender gap percentage in fully active life expectancy at age 65 was negative

FIGURE 2. Gender Gap Percentage in Fully Active Life Expectancy (FALE) at Age 65 (Years) and Gender Gap Percentage in Fully Active Life Expectancy (FALE) at Birth (Years), by Country

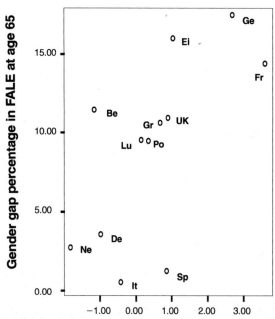

(Figure 3). Over the last twenty years, life expectancy in Denmark has not continued to increase as other European Union countries (Juel, Bjerregaard, and Madsen, 2000), and the trend in health expectancy has also differed between the sexes with men showing an overall gain and women a worsening of health (Bronnum-Hansen, 1998).

FIGURE 3. Gender Gap Percentage in Partly Active Life Expectancy (PALE) at Age 65 (Years) and Gender Gap Percentage in Life Expectancy (LE) at Age 65 (Years), by Country

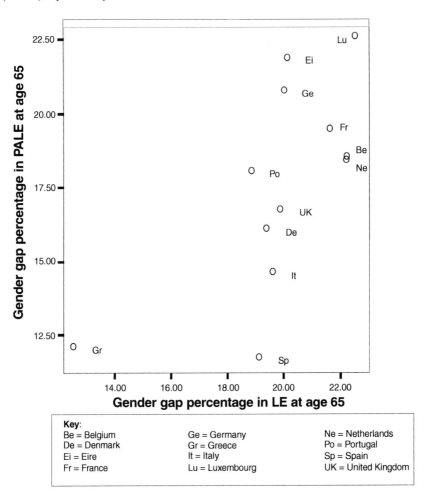

Although the ECHP goes a long way to collecting comparable disability data across European countries, a number of problems still remain. The major ones are the differing, and in some cases low, response rates between the countries, exclusion of the population within institutional care and the form of the disability question itself. The ECHP selects households for surveying, and in the 1994 wave the response rate for households varied from 35.8% (Luxembourg) to 90.1% (Greece), with a further 3 countries having response rates over 85% (Belgium, Italy, The Netherlands), and an overall average response rate of 74.4%. However, the response rate by country did not appear to be associated with health expectancies at birth or in later life, although a fuller analysis investigating possible gender differentials in response should be made.

In our calculations, as in many other health expectancy calculations, we have had to make assumptions about the population in institutional care, specifically that years of life lived with and without disability are in the same proportion for community-dwelling and institutional residents alike. Definitions, and therefore the prevalence of people in institutional care, differ across European countries. Proportions of the overall population in institutional care in 1995 varied from 12% in Belgium to 1% in Denmark, with the majority of countries being in the 3-6% range. The effect on the disability rates reported by the ECHP are difficult to predict, although when the institutionalization rate is high, the selection criteria are likely to be unselective and our assumption is likely to be reasonable. However, where institutionalization rates are extremely low, it is likely that admission criteria are highly selective and will result in a concentration of highly dependent people within institutions and a less dependent population outside. There was no evidence from our results that institutional rate was associated with lower or higher life expectancies or disability-free life expectancies in men or women. To fully understand the differences between European countries in disability-free life expectancy, prevalence of disability must explicitly include people within institutions in the same manner across countries.

Due to the large amount of information collected by the ECHP, the space available for health and disability items is small. It is, therefore, perhaps more important that the question or questions really reflect the needs of the users and are strongly linked to an underlying conceptual framework to ensure a true basis for translation. The current question is aimed at later in the disablement process, tapping activity restriction (Wood, 1975). However, it attempts to pick up lower levels of restriction through the responses of "Yes, severely," "Yes, to some extent," "No."

There may well be some gender differences in admission of severe activity restriction and that these differ also between cultures and, therefore, countries. A better method of increasing the range of severity detected would be to include functional limitation items, aimed at the body level, that would be less likely to be culturally and gender biased.

When disability at all levels of severity was used, the percentage difference in disability-free life expectancy for women over men at age 65 was positively associated with the percentage difference in disability-free life expectancy between birth and age 65, suggesting that values at younger ages may continue through to later life. This confirms other research that has found that poorer health in childhood increases ill-health in later life (van de Mheen, Stronks, Looman, and Mackenbach, 1998; Blackwell, Hayward, and Crimmins, 2001). However, the variation explained by our regression models was just under 50% suggesting that there are other factors determining the substantial variation in gender differences in health expectancies across European countries, though our study is not sufficient in its design to confirm this. Moreover, we found no clear evidence of any geographical patterns in the gender differentials either.

Differences in disability-free life expectancies between socio-economic groupings as well as levels of education have been found (Valkonen, Sihvonen, and Lahelma, 1994; Sihvonen et al., 1998; Bronnum-Hansen, 2000; Melzer et al., 2000) with more disadvantaged individuals experiencing shorter disability-free lives. Inequalities in health have been found within eastern European countries to be more strongly related to education than to socio-economic differences (Marmot and Bobak, 2000) although differences between western and eastern Europe are much greater than differences within the western European countries considered in our study. Clearer differences between men and women exist across Europe with regard to lifestyle factors and health behaviours and beliefs. Southern European countries tend to have a smaller proportion of women who smoke whilst in Denmark, smoking rates in women are the highest and still increasing (Hill, 1992). However, southern Europeans, particularly older and less educated individuals, report lower levels of physical activity and less belief in the need for exercise compared to the Finns who have experienced widespread health education and interventions on such benefits, particularly to cardiovascular health (Kafatos et al., 1999). A further difference between the northern and southern European countries concerns diet and the generally held views of the benefits to health of the Mediterranean diet, high in olive oil, vegetables, and fruit. In a study between the

United Kingdom and France, women were found to have healthier diets than men (Holdsworth et al., 2000). However, evidence is emerging that adolescents in southern Europe may be changing their diets for ones higher in saturated fats and carbohydrates (Cruz, 2000), with a possible future effect on health and longevity.

As mortality rates, particularly in men, continue to decline within most European countries, information to assist policy-makers in planning for the growing ageing populations is urgently needed. Although it is often noted that women live longer lives though generally in poorer health than their male counterparts, there has not been a full exploration of the reasons for these gender differences. The variability in the gender differences that we have found between the European populations, at first sight a relatively homogeneous population, together with information on health beliefs and practices should provide some insight into the mechanisms driving the differences. The continuing collection of truly comparable health and health-related data across Europe will provide countries with an opportunity to learn from each other's successes in order to maximize the health of older women and men in the future.

REFERENCES

Blackwell, D.L., Hayward, M.D., & Crimmins, E.M. (2001). Does childhood health affect chronic morbidity in later life? *Social Science and Medicine*, 52, 1269-1284.

Bone, M., Bebbington, R., Jagger, C., Morgan, K., & Nicolaas, N. (1995). *Health Expectancy and Its Uses*. London: HMSO.

Bronnum-Hansen, H. (1998). Trends in health expectancy in Denmark, 1987-1994. *Danish Medical Bulletin*, 45(2), 217-221.

Bronnum-Hansen, H. (2000). Socioeconomic differences in health expectancy in Denmark. *Scandinavian Journal of Public Health*, 28(3), 194-199.

Cruz, J.A.A. (2000). Dietary habits and nutritional status in adolescents over Europe-Southern Europe. *European Journal of Clinical Nutrition*, 54, 29-35.

Eurostat. (1996). *The European Community Household Panel (ECHP): Survey methodology and implementation*. Eurostat: Volume 1.

Hill, C. (1992). Trends in tobacco use in Europe. Journal of the National Cancer Institute. *Monographs*, 12, 21-24.

Holdsworth, M., Gerber, M., Haslam, C., Scali, J., Bearsdworth, A., Avallone, M.H., & Sherratt, E. (2000). A comparison of dietary behaviour in Central England and a French Mediterranean region. *European Journal of Clinical Nutrition*, 54, 530-539.

Juel, K., Bjerregaard, P., & Madsen, M. (2000). Mortality and life expectancy in Denmark and in other European countries. *European Journal of Public Health*, 10, 93-100.

Kafatos, A., Manios, Y., Markatji, I., Giachetti, I., Vaz de Almeida, M.D., & Engstrom, L.M. (1999). Regional, demographic and national influences on attitudes and beliefs with regard to physical activity, body weight and health in a nationally representative sample in the European Union. *Public Health Nutrition*, 2(1A), 87-95.

Marmot, M., & Bobak, M. (2000). International comparators and poverty and health in Europe. *British Medical Journal*, 321, 1124-1128.

Melzer, D., McWilliams, B., Brayne, C., Johnson, T., & Bond, J. (2000). Socioeconomic status and the expectation of disability in old age: Estimates for England. *Journal of Epidemiology & Community Health*, 54(4), 286-292.

Perenboom, R.J., Boshuizen, H.C., & van de Water, H.P. (1993). Trends in health expectancies in the Netherlands, 1981-1990. In J.M. Robine, C.D. Mathers, M.R. Bone, & I. Romieu (Eds.), *Calculation of health expectancies: Harmonization, consensus achieved and future perspectives*. Montrouge: John Libbey Eurotext.

Robine, J.M., & Mormiche, P. (1994). Estimation de la valeur de l'espérance de vie sans incapacitié en France en 1991 et élaboration de séries chronologiques. *Solidarité Santé*, 1, 17-36.

Robine, J.M., Romieu, I., & Cambois, E. (1999). Health expectancy indicators. *Bulletin of the World Health Organization*, 77(2), 181-185.

Romieu, I., & Robine, J.M. (1994). World atlas on health expectancy calculations. In C.D. Mathers, J. McCallum, & J.M. Robine (Eds.), *Advances in health expectancies*. Canberra: Australian Institute of Health and Welfare, AGPS.

Sihvonen, A.P., Kunst, A.E., Lahelma, E., Valkonen, T., & Mackenbach, J.P. (1998). Socioeconomic inequalities in health expectancy in Finland and Norway in the late 1980s. *Social Science & Medicine*, 47(3), 303-315.

Sullivan, D.F. (1971). A single index of mortality and morbidity. *HSMHA Health Report*, 86, 347-354.

Trichopoulou, A., & Vasilopoulou, E. (2000). Mediterranean diet and longevity. *British Journal of Nutrition*, 84, S205-S209.

Valkonen, T., Sihvonen, A-P., & Lahelma, E. (1994). Disability-free life expectancy by level of education in Finland. In: C.D. Mathers, J. McCallum, & J.M. Robine (Eds.), *Advances in Health Expectancies*. Canberra: Australian Institute of Health and Welfare, AGPS.

van Ginneken, J.K., Dissevelt, A.G., van de Water, H.P., & van Sonsbeek, J.L. (1991). Results of two methods to determine health expectancy in The Netherlands in 1981-1985. *Social Science & Medicine*, 32(10), 1129-1136.

van de Mheen, H., Stronks, K., Looman, C.W.N., & Mackenbach, J.P. (1998). Role of childhood health in the explanation of socioeconomic inequalities in early adult health. *Journal of Epidemiology and Community Health*, 52, 15-19.

Van Oyen, H., Tafforeau, J., & Roelands, M. (1996). Regional inequities in health expectancy in Belgium. *Social Science & Medicine*, 43(11), 1673-1678.

Verbrugge, L.M. (1997). A global disability indicator. *Journal of Aging Studies*, 11, 337-362.

Health Expectancies in Japan:
Gender Differences
and Policy Implications for Women

Ichiro Tsuji, MD
Catherine Sauvaget, MD
Shigeru Hisamichi, MD

SUMMARY. Based on prospective observation of elderly people in the community in Japan, we compared the time-course of development and progression of physical disability between women and men. Men experienced disability at a younger age and at a faster rate than did women. The duration of time spent with disability in women was twice as long as in men. Consequently, women consume about two-thirds of the total resources of formal caregiving services in Japan. Women in Japan are increasingly educated, postponing marriage to higher ages, and less likely to care for parents in the home. Given these changes in family structure and

Ichiro Tsuji, Catherine Sauvaget, and Shigeru Hisamichi are affiliated with the Department of Public Health, Tohoku University School of Medicine, Sendai, Japan. Catherine Sauvaget is also affiliated with the Department of Epidemiology, Radiation Effect Research Foundation, Hiroshima, Japan.

Address correspondence to: Ichiro Tsuji, MD, Department of Public Health, Tohoku University School of Medicine, 2-1 Seiryo-machi, Aoba-ku, Sendai, 980-8575 Japan (E-Mail: tsuji1@mail.cc.tohoku.ac.jp).

The authors are grateful to Drs. Yumi Hashizume and Midori Ashida for their valuable suggestions and insights. This study was in part supported by a research grant from the Japanese Ministry of Health, Labour, and Welfare.

135

social norms, the capacity for informal family caregiving has decreased dramatically. A recently enacted national long-term care insurance system may further change the picture of caregiving. *[Article copies available for a fee from The Haworth Document Delivery Service: 1-800-HAWORTH. E-mail address: <getinfo@haworthpressinc.com> Website: <http://www. HaworthPress.com> © 2002 by The Haworth Press, Inc. All rights reserved.]*

KEYWORDS. Active life expectancy, activities of daily living (ADL), instrumental activities of daily living (IADL), prospective study, long-term care insurance, Japan

POPULATION AGING IN JAPAN

Over the last half of the 20th century, the population in Japan aged at a faster pace than in any other country. In 1950, only 4.1 million Japanese (4.9% of the population) were aged 65 years or older. In 2000, the number of the aged population increased by more than five times, to 21.9 million (17.2% of the population). This percentage is among the highest in the world. It is estimated that, in the year 2015, one out of four Japanese people will be 65 years of age or older (Ministry of Health and Welfare, 2000a).

This drastic change in the demography in Japanese society is partly attributable to a rapid increase in life expectancy. In the early 20th century, Japanese people had a shorter life expectancy than people in other industrialized countries. For instance, the life expectancy for Japanese women born in 1926-30 was 46.5 years, compared to 61 years for American women born in 1929-31, 62.9 years for British women born in 1930-32, 58.8 years for German women born in 1924-26, and 59 years for French women born in 1928-33. After World War II, however, the life expectancy of Japanese people increased at a faster rate than in any other country. Now, the life expectancy of Japanese people is the longest in the world: 84.3 years for women and 77.6 years for men born in 1999 (Ministry of Health and Welfare, 2000a).

The World Health Organization (WHO, 2000) reported that the healthy life expectancy of Japanese people was also the longest among the WHO member states. Disability Adjusted Life Expectancy (DALE), defined as the expected number of years to be lived in what might be termed the equivalent of "full health," was 77.2 years for women and 71.9 years for Japanese men in 1999. The difference between the total life expectancy and the DALE could be considered as the expected number of life-years to be spent with disability or ill-health. For Japanese women, the duration was 7.1 years, rated the 27th shortest in the world. For Japanese men, it was 5.7 years and the 17th shortest. The increase in healthy life expectancy in Japanese people was not accompanied by a longer period of life with disability. However, we are not without problems. As the population ages, the number of frail or disabled people is rapidly increasing. At the same time, because of changing family structures and social norms, the capacity for informal caregiving within the family is rapidly decreasing in Japan.

In this article, we present data for active life expectancy (ALE) of older Japanese people based on our longitudinal observations, which show gender differences in development and progression of disabilities in later life. We discuss how both the demographic structure and the traditional social norms for caregiving are changing rapidly in Japan, and finally, introduce the long-term care insurance (LTCI) recently established by the Japanese government.

COMPARISON OF ACTIVE LIFE EXPECTANCY (ALE) BETWEEN MEN AND WOMEN

Study 1: Gender Difference in Life Years With and Without Disability

The purpose of this prospective study was to compare ALE between women and men. We followed the physical functioning status of aged people living in Sendai City, Japan, for three years and calculated the ALE (Tsuji et al., 1995). We conducted a baseline survey in October 1988 on 3,704 subjects, a 5% random sample of residents aged 65 years and over in Sendai. The questionnaires were hand-delivered and collected at the subjects' residences by trained survey personnel. The subjects were asked to complete the questionnaire regarding demographics, the ability to perform activities of daily living (ADLs), and medical history. The overall response rate was 93% (N = 3,459).

A follow-up survey was conducted three years later in October 1991. During these three years, 75 subjects (2%) left the city, and 352 (10%) died. Of the remaining 3,032 subjects, 2,759 (91%) responded to the follow-up survey.

In calculating the ALE, we classified the subjects as dependent or inactive if they required assistance to perform at least one of the following

ADLs: bathing, dressing, toileting, and eating. The subjects who were able to perform all these tasks by themselves were classified as independent or active. We calculated age- and sex-specific transition probabilities between the baseline and the follow-up surveys by a person-year method; from independence to dependence, from independence to death, from dependence to independence, and from dependence to death. With these transition probabilities, we constructed a single-year increment-decrement life table to calculate the ALE, which was defined as the number of years a subject at a given age is expected to live without disability in performing basic ADLs (Branch et al., 1991).

Table 1 indicates total life expectancy (TLE), ALE, and years to be spent with disability for women and men. At age 65 years, TLE was 20.4 years for women and 16.1 years for men. ALE at age 65 was 17.7 years for women and 14.7 years for men. Although ALE was longer for women than for men, active life occupied a smaller proportion of total life for women (86.8%) than for men (91.3%). Among those aged 77 years or older, TLE for men at a given age was as long as ALE for women at corresponding ages.

The duration to be spent with disability was 2.7 years for women and 1.4 years for men. Although both TLE and ALE decreased with age, the duration to be spent with disability was relatively constant over the ages. It ranged from 2.5 to 2.9 years for women, and from 1.1 to 1.4 years for men. The gender difference in the number of years to be spent with disability was about two-fold.

Study 2: Gender Differences in Progress of Disability

The purpose of this study was to clarify gender differences regarding development and progression of disability in later life. We measured disability-free expectancy according to three functional levels: basic ADLs, instrumental ADLs (IADLs), and locomotion (Sauvaget et al., 1999). We conducted a baseline survey in September 1994 on all 3,590 residents aged 65 years and over in Wakuya Town, Japan. Wakuya is a typical rural area where the main industry is agriculture.

The baseline survey was made with a self-completed questionnaire. Members of the Health Promotion Committee of the town visited the subjects, asked them to complete the questionnaire, then collected the questionnaire about a week later. The questionnaire included items regarding demographics, the ability to perform basic ADLs (bathing, dressing, transferring from a bed to a chair, and eating), the ability to perform IADLs (shopping for daily necessities, preparing meals, and

TABLE 1. Total Life Expectancy, Active Life Expectancy, and Years with Disability According to Sex and Age.

Age	Men				Women		
	TLE	ALE	Disability		TLE	ALE	Disability
65	16.1	14.7	1.4		20.4	17.7	2.7
66	15.3	14.1	1.2		19.5	16.7	2.8
67	14.8	13.5	1.3		18.6	15.9	2.7
68	13.9	12.7	1.2		17.8	15.3	2.5
69	13.2	12.1	1.1		17.2	14.3	2.9
70	12.6	11.2	1.4		16.4	13.6	2.8
71	11.7	10.8	0.9		15.6	12.8	2.8
72	11.1	9.9	1.2		15.0	12.1	2.9
73	10.4	9.3	1.1		14.0	11.5	2.5
74	9.7	8.6	1.1		13.3	10.6	2.7
75	9.0	7.9	1.1		12.5	9.8	2.7
76	8.7	7.5	1.2		11.7	9.1	2.6
77	8.3	7.0	1.3		11.0	8.4	2.6
78	7.8	6.2	1.6		10.2	7.6	2.6
79	7.2	5.5	1.7		9.4	7.2	2.2
80	6.4	5.2	1.2		9.0	6.6	2.4
81	6.1	4.8	1.3		8.3	6.0	2.3
82	5.7	4.3	1.4		7.8	5.9	1.9
83	5.1	3.7	1.4		7.7	5.3	2.4
84	4.7	3.3	1.4		6.9	4.6	2.3
85	4.7	3.3	1.4		6.2	4.1	2.1
86	4.4	2.9	1.5		6.0	3.8	2.2
87	4.1	3.3	0.8		5.6	4.0	1.6
88	3.8	3.2	0.6		4.9	3.4	1.5
89	3.8	3.2	0.6		4.2	2.7	1.5
90	3.5	3.1	0.4		3.7	2.7	1.0

TLE: total life expectancy (yr)
ALE: active life expectancy (yr)
Disability: years to be spent with disability (yr)

managing money), and the ability to perform locomotor activities (walking 50 meters and climbing a flight of stairs). In this questionnaire, the items on basic ADLs and locomotion were adopted from the Barthel ADL Index (Mahoney and Barthel, 1965), and those on IADLs were adopted from the instrumental self-maintenance scale developed by the Tokyo Metropolitan Institute of Gerontology (Koyano et al., 1991).

For the baseline survey, the overall response rate was 90.1% (N = 3,235). We conducted a follow-up survey two years later in September 1996. During this period, 26 subjects (1%) left the town and 225 (7%) died. Of the remaining 2,984 subjects, 2,936 (98%) responded.

We calculated the ALE with a single-year increment-decrement life table for each of the three functional levels: basic ADLs, IADLs, and locomotion. We defined the subjects as dependent or inactive if they required assistance in performing one or more tasks at a given functional level. In this report, ALE in basic ADLs is defined as the number of years a subject at a given age is expected to live without disability in performing basic ADLs. ALE in IADLs is defined as the number of years to be spent without disability in IADLs, and ALE in locomotion as the duration without disability for locomotor functions.

The prevalence of disability in basic ADLs was 9.3% for women and 9.5% for men in the 1994 baseline survey. For IADLs, it was 22.2% in women and 19.8% in men. For locomotion, it was 8.4% in women and 5.9% in men. The age-adjusted prevalence rate of either level of disability was not significantly different between the genders. Table 2 shows TLE, ALE, and duration of life with disability in basic ADLs, IADLs, and locomotion, respectively, for every five years of age and sex. At age 65, TLE was 17.1 years for women and 13.8 years for men. For basic ADLs, women were expected to live without disability for 16.0 years (93.6% of the total life) and with disability for 1.1 years. For men, it was estimated to be 13.2 years (95.7%) and 0.6 years, respectively. The duration to be spent with disability for women was about twice as long as that for men, which was consistent with the results for Study 1.

For IADLs, ALE was 12.9 years (75.6% of the total life) for women and 10.9 years (79.1%) for men. The duration to be spent with disability in IADLs was 4.2 years for women and 2.9 years for men. For locomotor activity, the duration without disability was 14.7 years (86.0% of the total life) for women and 13.2 years (95.7%) for men. The duration to be spent with disability in locomotor activities was 2.4 years in women and 0.6 years in men. The difference in the length of time with a locomotor disability between women and men was four-fold.

The time-course of development and progression of physical disability was clearly different between women and men. The average woman at age 65 would live fully independent for 12.9 years. She would then live with IADL disability, but without disability in basic ADLs and locomotion, for 1.8 years. This period would be followed by another 1.3 years with disability in both IADLs and locomotion. The final 1.1 years of life would be spent dependent in all three physical functions. Out of a

TABLE 2. Total Life Expectancy, Active Life Expectancy, and Duration with Disability in Basic ADL, Instrumental ADL, and Mobility According to Sex and Age

	Basic ADL				IADL		Mobility	
Age	TLE	ALE	Disability		ALE	Disability	ALE	Disability
				Men				
65	13.8	13.2	0.6		10.9	2.9	13.2	0.6
70	10.1	9.6	0.5		7.7	2.4	9.6	0.5
75	7.3	6.8	0.5		5.1	2.2	6.7	0.6
80	5.4	4.7	0.7		3.0	2.4	4.6	0.8
85	3.1	2.5	0.6		0.5	2.6	2.2	0.9
				Women				
65	17.1	16.0	1.1		12.9	4.2	14.7	2.4
70	14.3	13.1	1.2		9.8	4.5	11.7	2.6
75	10.0	8.9	1.1		6.0	4.0	7.6	2.4
80	6.7	5.6	1.1		3.2	3.5	4.6	2.1
85	2.8	2.0	0.8		0.9	1.9	1.7	1.1

TLE: total life expectancy (yr)
ALE: active life expectancy (yr)
Disability: years to be spent with disability (yr)
ADL: activity of daily living

total life expectancy of 13.8 years, men at age 65 were expected to live for 10.9 years without any functional disability, then become IADL disabled. The state of being dependent in IADLs but independent in basic ADLs and locomotion would last for 2.3 years. Men would then become disabled in basic ADLs and locomotion at almost the same time. Finally, they would die within 0.6 years of becoming dependent in all three physical functions.

These results indicated that there is a sequential order in development of physical disabilities in later life. Among a variety of physical functions, an earlier decline was observed in tasks related to IADLs, followed by a decline in basic ADLs. Thus, in both genders, ALE for IADLs was shorter than the ALEs for basic ADLs and locomotion. There was a marked gender difference in the process of developing and progressing disability (disablement process). Men experienced disability at a younger age and at a faster rate than did women. Another gender difference in the disablement process was that a disability in basic ADLs and a disability in locomotion developed almost simultaneously in men while there was a time lag of about 0.7 years for women between the onset of a disability in locomotion and that in basic ADLs.

This gender difference in the disablement process could be attributable in part to the difference between women and men in diseases responsible for development and progression of disability (Sauvaget et al., 1999). In the baseline survey, self-reported histories of arthritis and osteoporosis were significantly more prevalent in women (M:F = 1:3.6, $p < 0.001$ and M:F = 1:4.8, $p < 0.001$, respectively). Among those who developed a disability in basic ADLs during the follow-up, stroke incidence was significantly higher by 2.8 times in men, and heart disease was 7.4 times higher. The gender difference in prevalence and incidence of diseases responsible for disability in these subjects is similar to those in other population-based surveys in Japan. Surveys of the older people living in five communities in Japan indicated that histories of fracture and neuralgia were more prevalent in women, and those of diabetes and stroke were more prevalent in men (Kishimoto et al., 1998). The impact of stroke on development of disability among older people was reported to be different between women and men. According to a longitudinal study on a probability sample of the Japanese population, the population-attributable risk percent of cerebrovascular diseases causing disability in basic ADLs was as high as 54.0% in men but only 21.7% in women (Hayakawa et al., 2001). In conclusion, the etiological mechanisms of physical disability are different between women and men. Stroke and its risk factors are more likely for elderly men, resulting in an acute deterioration of physical functioning and a relatively short time spent with disability. Stroke usually affects the ability to perform basic ADLs and locomotor activities at the same time, so the time-course of the disablement process in men seems quite plausible. On the other hand, the impact of osteoporotic and arthritic conditions would be greater for elderly women, resulting in a slow progress of disability and a longer time spent with disability.

JAPANESE WOMEN AS CARE RECEIVERS

The gender difference in the duration to be spent with disability produces corresponding gender differences in the needs and demands for caregiving. The product of the number of people at a given age and the number of years to be spent with disability for this age represents the sum of the person-years to be spent with disability by all the people in this cohort throughout their lives. According to the 1995 Census of Japan, 712,209 women (52%) and 648,860 men (48%) were 65 years old. According to the results of study 2, the time they are expected to be living with disability in basic ADLs was estimated to be 1.1 years for women and 0.6 years for men. Therefore, the total person-years to be spent with disability by the whole population in this birth cohort would be 783,430 person-years for women and 389,316 person-years for men. Of the total need for caregiving, 1,172,446 person-years, women consume 67% and men consume only 33%.

Overall, the national statistics of Japan indicate that the majority of the people who receive formal caregiving services are women. According to the Ministry of Health and Welfare of Japan (1997a), a total of 232,000 people in Japan used formal home care services in 1994. Of those, women constituted 64%. Among 390,000 day care users, 71% were women. Of 119,000 people who ever used respite care, 61% were women. About two out of three nursing home residents in Japan were women (Ministry of Health and Welfare, 2000b). In conclusion, the majority of care receivers in Japan are women.

JAPANESE WOMEN AS CAREGIVERS

In addition to the fact that the majority of care receivers in Japan are women, the majority of caregivers in Japan are also women. Most survey results in Japan agreed that approximately 80% of family caregivers are women. According to a survey (Ministry of Health and Welfare, 1997b) asking next of kin who looked after the decedents aged 65 years and over (N = 3,130) in Japan in 1995, the wife was the most common caregiver, constituting 31.6% of the total caregivers. The next most common caregivers were the wife of the eldest son (27.6%), or a daughter (20.0%). In this survey, about 35% of female caregivers reported that they had resigned from a job for family caregiving.

This emphasis on women as family caregivers reflects the traditional social norms of Japan. Under the traditional norms, Japanese women were expected to obey and respect men, to stay at home for housekeeping rather than to work outside the home, and to be fully responsible for taking care of children and elderly parents-in-law (Sodei, 1995; Hashizume, 2000). Under this tradition, the eldest or first-born son is the "leader" of the family system, and elderly parents ought to live with the eldest son's family. A three-generation family home was the most common place for elderly parents to live. The wife of the eldest son is regarded as being fully responsible for taking care of her parents-in-law.

Many people feel it is a stigma to place a parent in a nursing home, and feel reluctant to have service providers come into their homes. Consequently, informal support within the family was the main resource for taking care of frail or disabled elderly people in Japan (Sodei, 1995; Hashizume, 2000).

JAPANESE SOCIETY AND CULTURE IN TRANSITION

With the rapid westernization of the Japanese lifestyle over the past 50 years, gender expectations have also changed. For instance, an increasing number of women receive higher education. In 1960, only 5.5% of female high school graduates attended college or higher level education, compared with 14.9% of men. In 2000, 48.7% of girls and 49.4% of boys went on to higher education (Ministry of Education and Culture, 2000). The gender difference has disappeared. An increasing number of Japanese women choose to work outside rather than to stay at home.

With this trend, the traditional differentiation of gender roles in Japan has been disappearing. These changes have resulted in drastic transitions in demography, such as postponement of marriage to an older age, a decrease in the number of childbirths, and changes in the family structure. First, the mean age at the first marriage for Japanese women increased from 22.9 years in 1950 to 26.3 years in 1995. Only 5.7% of Japanese women remained unmarried until 30 years of age in 1950, while the figure increased to 19.7% in 1995 (Ministry of Health and Welfare, 2000a). Second, the total fertility rate decreased from 3.65 in 1950 to 1.34 in 1999, and is now among the lowest in the world (Ministry of Health and Welfare, 2000a). Third, the family structure has been changing rapidly in Japan. The three-generation family has been decreasing, and the most common type of household is now a nuclear family, occupying 60% of the total households in Japan in 1999. Among the households with members aged 65 years and over, the three-generation family decreased from 54.4% in 1975 to 27.3% in 1999. In contrast, the proportion of older people living alone increased from 8.6% in 1975 to 18.2% in 1999 (Ministry of Health and Welfare, 2000a).

All these demographic transitions in Japan resulted in a lower capacity for informal caregiving within the family. The rapid changes are occurring not only in demographics but also in social norms. Our way of life and thinking also are rapidly shifting from the traditional Asian values to westernized ones. Because these changes are taking place so fast, we may say that the different generations have different value systems. Older people grew up under the strong influence of the traditional values. Younger people feel that these values are obsolete. Middle-aged people may understand both sets of values, and they are actually feeling that they are like a pendulum swinging back and forth between the two distinct value systems. Indeed, Sodei (1995) reported that most Japanese women aged in their 50s or 60s, who were taking care of their mothers-in-law, thought that they could not expect their children or daughters-in-law to take care of them when they were older.

Now, the number of the frail or disabled elderly is steadily increasing because of the rapid aging of the Japanese population. The number of ambulatory but frail elderly people is estimated to be 1.3 million in 2000. This figure is estimated to double, to 2.6 million, by 2025. Similarly, the number of bedridden elderly is projected to increase from 1.2 million in 2000 to 2.3 million in 2025 (Ministry of Health and Welfare, 2000a). The demand for caregiving is escalating. However, with the changes in family structure and social norms, the capacity for informal caregiving within a family system is decreasing dramatically. The traditional system of caregiving in Japan is in crisis, which led us to establish national long-term care insurance in April of 2000.

LONG-TERM CARE INSURANCE IN JAPAN

The long-term care insurance (LTCI) is a mandatory social insurance that covers almost all formal caregiving services for elderly people in Japan (Ministry of Health and Welfare, 2000c; Campbell & Ikegami, 2000). Everyone aged 40 years and over in Japan must pay insurance premiums, the amount being dependent on income level. Services under LTCI are available to all people aged 65 years and over, as well as individuals aged between 40 and 64 years who have an age-related disability such as stroke, Parkinson's disease, chronic obstructive pulmonary disease, and so forth.

When an individual applies for services to the municipal government, service personnel assess the applicant's mental and physical conditions using an 85-item assessment form. Based on this assessment, a government-made computer program determines the eligibility level for the person, out of six service levels. These six service levels are determined with the amount of time required each day for caregiving, as well as the monetary value that an individual at a given service level may consume for formal services under LTCI per month, ranging from

61,500 Japanese yen (US$ 512) to 358,000 Japanese yen (US$ 2,983). The price of each service is determined by the government. An applicant then chooses services within a monetary value limit for his/her own service level. A care manager, who is licensed by the government, assists the applicant to make better decisions and provides a care plan (weekly schedule of services). The service eligibility and the care plan will be revised every six months. A recipient of the services is required to pay 10% of the services charges as a co-payment. Formal caregiving services include both institutional care and community-based care. The institutional care includes three different types of institutions: a nursing home, which provides caregiving services in ADLs; a health facility for the elderly, which is an intermediate facility that provides functional rehabilitation as well as caregiving; and a long-term care ward in a hospital, which provides medical care for disabled patients at a chronic stage of illness. Community-based care includes services such as caregiving and housekeeping at home, a bathing service, nursing care at home, functional training at home, day care services, respite care at institutions, a group home for the demented elderly, and reconstruction of houses.

Since the program started in April of 2000, no formal statistics on utilization and expenditures on LTCI are available. The government estimated that 2.7 million elderly people, or 12.4%, are eligible to use the services in 2000, and that only one-third of the eligible people living at home would actually use the services because some people are still reluctant to have somebody in their home to provide care. It is estimated that the total expenditures in the first year would be 4.8 trillion Japanese yen (approximately 40 million US dollars). The utilization rate would then increase, and estimated expenditure at maturity, eight or ten years later, when 80% of eligible elderly people at home use the benefits, would be 7.0 trillion Japanese yen (approximately 58 million US dollars).

PERSPECTIVES OF AGING AND CAREGIVING IN JAPAN

The changes in family structure and social norms in Japan caused a decrease in the capacity for informal caregiving. LTCI would further change people's attitudes about formal caregiving services. Because everyone pays premiums for LTCI, people may become more willing to use formal caregiving. Together with the decreasing capacity for family caregiving and the increasing number of frail or disabled elderly, the demand for formal care services is likely to increase quickly in Japan.

In the meantime, gender differences in active life expectancy will have differential impacts on the need for formal caregiving services between men and women. Because active life expectancy is shorter in men than in women, men are most likely to be cared for by their spouse. On the other hand, because the active life expectancy of women is longer than the total life expectancy of men, women are most likely to become disabled after their spouse dies. Under the circumstance where the capacity for family caregiving is decreasing, most women would receive care from someone other than a spouse.

The changes in family structure and social norms will affect women more deeply than men. Women may become more dependent upon formal caregiving services and, consequently, put a heavy burden on LTCI finances and other social security resources. It is urgently required that we establish comprehensive measures toward preventing or postponing the onset of disability, especially for women.

REFERENCES

Branch, L.G., Guralnik, J.M., Foley, D.J. et al. (1991). Active life expectancy for 10,000 Caucasian men and women in three communities. J Gerontol, 46, M145-50.

Campbell, J.J., & Ikegami, N. (2000). Long-term care insurance comes to Japan. Health Affairs, 19, 26-39.

Hashizume, Y. (2000). Gender issues and Japanese family-centered caregiving for frail elderly parents of parents-in-law in modern Japan: From the sociocultural and historical perspectives. Public Health Nursing, 17, 25-31.

Hayakawa, T., Okayama, A., Ueshima, H., Kita, Y., Choudhury, S.R., & Tamaki, J. (2001). Prevalence of impaired activities of daily living and impact of stroke and lower limb fracture on it in Japanese elderly people. CVD Prevention (in print).

Kishimoto, M., Ojima, T., Nakamura, Y., Yanagawa, H., Fujita, Y. et al. (1998). Relationship between the level of activities of daily living and chronic medical conditions among the elderly. J Epidemiol, 8, 272-277.

Koyano, W., Shibata, H., Nakazato, K. et al. (1991). Measurement of competence: Reliability and validity of the TMIG index of competence. Arch Gerontol Geriatr, 13, 103-116.

Mahoney, F.I., & Barthel, D.W. (1965). Functional evaluation: The Barthel Index. Maryland, St Med J, 14, 61-65.

Ministry of Education and Culture, Japan. (2000). Wagakunino Bunkyo Sesaku 2000 [Educational and Cultural Policy in Japan 2000]. (In Japanese) Printing Bureau, Ministry of Finance, Tokyo.

Ministry of Health and Welfare, Japan. (1997a). Kenkou Fukushi Kanren Service Juyou Jittai Chosa 1994 [Survey on Demands for Health and Welfare Services]. (In Japanese) Health and Welfare Statistics Association, Tokyo.

Ministry of Health and Welfare, Japan. (1997b). Report on the Socioeconomic Survey of Vital Statistics: Deaths of the Aged 1995. (In Japanese with English summary) Health and Welfare Statistics Association, Tokyo.

Ministry of Health and Welfare, Japan. (2000a). Statistical Abstracts on Health and Welfare in Japan 2000. Health and Welfare Statistics Association, Tokyo.

Ministry of Health and Welfare, Japan. (2000b). Shakai Shisetsu Tou Chosa Houkoku 1999 [Survey Report on Social Institutions]. (In Japanese) Health and Welfare Statistics Association, Tokyo.

Ministry of Health and Welfare, Japan. (2000c). Annual Reports on Health and Welfare 1998-1999: Social Security and National Life (http://www.mhlw.go.jp/english/wp/wp-hw/index.html)

Sauvaget, C., Tsuji, I., Aonuma, T., & Hisamichi, S. (1999). Health-life expectancy according to various functional levels. J Am Geriatr Soc, 47, 1326-1331.

Sodei, T. (1995). Care of the Elderly: A Woman's Issue. In K. Fujimura-Fanselow & A. Kameda (Eds.) Japanese Women: New Feminist Perspectives on the Past, Present, and Future. New York, The Feminist Press.

Tsuji, I., Minami, Y., Fukao, A., Hisamichi, S., Asano, H., & Sato, M. (1995). Active life expectancy among the elderly Japanese. J Gerontol, 50A, M173-M176.

World Health Organization. (2000). Healthy Life Expectancy Rankings: Based on the World Health Organization's Disability Adjusted Life Expectancy (DALE). WHO Statistical Information System (WHOSIS) (*http://www-nt.who.int/whosis/statistics/*)

Disability Among Older Women and Men in Fiji: Concerns for the Future

Sela V. Panapasa, PhD

SUMMARY. This study examines the composition of elderly population at risk of disability and speculates the impact of disability on the quality of their lives and their longevity. Using census and survey data collected in Fiji, life table estimates of unimpaired life expectancy across time are presented for older people and the potential costs of disability, in terms of productive years of life lost. From a planning perspective, the study discusses medical and support services that may be needed to support older individuals in Fiji. The study also describes policy implications of the findings, focusing on the older women, and considers the implications for older women of other developing countries. *[Article copies available for a fee from The Haworth Document Delivery Service: 1-800-HAWORTH. E-mail address: <getinfo@haworthpressinc.com> Website: <http://www.HaworthPress. com> © 2002 by The Haworth Press, Inc. All rights reserved.]*

Sela V. Panapasa is an NIA postdoctoral fellow at the Population Studies Center.

Address correspondence to: Sela V. Panapasa, PSC, Institute for Social Research, 426 Thompson Street, PO Box 1248, Ann Arbor, MI 48106.

Support for this research was provided by a Center grant from the National Institute on Aging (5T32AG0021).

The author would like to thank Timoci Bainimarama, Government Statistician of Fiji, for granting permission to use the 1996 Fiji Census; without his support this study would not have been possible.

[Haworth co-indexing entry note]: "Disability Among Older Women and Men in Fiji: Concerns for the Future." Panapasa, Sela V. Co-published simultaneously in *Journal of Women & Aging* (The Haworth Press, Inc.) Vol. 14, No. 1/2, 2002, pp. 149-162; and: *Health Expectations for Older Women: International Perspectives* (ed: Sarah B. Laditka) The Haworth Press, Inc., 2002, pp. 149-162. Single or multiple copies of this article are available for a fee from The Haworth Document Delivery Service [1-800-HAWORTH 9:00 a.m. - 5:00 p.m. (EST). E-mail address: getinfo@haworthpressinc.com].

KEYWORDS. Aging, disability, developing country, gender and health, Pacific Islands

INTRODUCTION

In the past two decades, Fiji has seen dramatic increases in both the proportional and numerical size of its older populations due to the combined impacts of declining fertility and rising life expectancy. These sudden increases raise concern for a number of issues related to the welfare of the elderly, including the treatment and costs involved with old age disability, and the level of care that can be reasonably provided to those who are physically impaired. Similarly, as the risk of disability and chronic illness is expected to grow rapidly with increased longevity, it is unclear whether the needs of the disabled elderly can be met by existing social systems.

The purpose of this study is to employ the limited data available on disability in Fiji to examine the composition of the elderly population at risk of disability and to speculate the impact of disability on the quality of their lives and their longevity. Using census and survey data, estimates of unimpaired life expectancy across time are presented for older people, as well as the risk of being impaired as of 1996. From a planning perspective, the study discusses medical and support services that may be needed to support other older individuals in Fiji. The study also describes policy implication of the findings focusing on older women and considers the implications for older women of other developing countries.

THEORETICAL BACKGROUND

The measurement of disability in the developing world is a topic of increasing interest in the research literature of aging in non-Western nations. While early research attempted to address this topic in terms of Western constructs such Activities of Daily Living (ADLs), increasingly gerontological research in the developing world is assuming a multidisciplinary approach that addresses disability in terms of context as well as diagnosed conditions (DaVanzo et al., 1994; Hermalin et al., 1996; Lewis, 1998; Rahman, 1999; Smith, 1994). This increasing emphasis on context grows from the recognition that the severity of impairment is impacted by a number of factors outside the traditional

Western medico-social support systems. These concepts, often encompassed under the theory of Social Constructionism, are centrally concerned with meaning and emphasize the crucial importance of learning from disabled people's experience to better understand disability within different cultural constructs (Oliver, 1998).

Lacking access to modern diagnostic and treatment regimens, the elderly in most developing nations continue to depend upon traditional approaches to maintenance and autonomy with the onset of disability. The need for a multidisciplinary approach towards understanding care issues is important as systems that improve the quality of life at older ages are typically interrelated. The lack of smooth pathways in many urban and rural areas, for example, simultaneously minimizes the value of wheelchairs and walkers and increases the risk of falls and injuries among the elderly.

These interrelated systems of care need to be addressed both at the community level and within the family if the elderly are to receive consistent levels of support services. A classic example being how basic necessities for a good diet or medication are tied to the overall family economy which in turn depends upon the economic stability of the community and its infrastructures. In the multigenerational households that remain the norm in most developing countries, the needs of the elderly must be evaluated within the household economies. In the face of limited resources, choices must be made as to who will receive access to specific goods and services. As the economic power of the household rarely resides in the hands of the elderly resident, it places them in a position of dependency in relation to the primary decision makers. When costs exceed family resources, care for the elderly may represent insurmountable barriers to families in the developing world (Barr, 1990; Bose, 1996).

Finally, systems of disability among the elderly need to be addressed in terms of *who* will pay for that care. In most developing nations, the direct cost of care is borne directly by the elderly individual and communally with the family of residence. Consequently, a calculus of care exists within the household in which the elderly live and the elderly must evaluate their need for care within the framework of that economy. If the elderly feel their need for care is reasonable and legitimate, they can negotiate for care, medication, or support with the decision makers of the household. The economic decision makers must then decide whether the request for care can be met within the overall needs and constraints of the household economy. This process of negotiation clearly translates into issues of household power and rank. An aging patriarchal household head, for example, would have much higher status and right to limited family resources than an elderly aunt taken in by a family due to systems of family obligation. Alternatively, the elderly with weaker bargaining power may simply dismiss disabling conditions as the product of "old age" as they recognize their limited ability to negotiate for care (Herzog et al., 1997; Smith, 1994; Weisner et al., 1977).

The problems of unmet need represent the greatest single barrier to improving the quality of life of the disabled elderly. This is driven by the fact that the majority of the elderly continue to reside in rural areas, thus limiting their access to and availability of medical services. The presence of a health care service infrastructure in urban areas clearly plays a role in minimizing the impacts of disability. With young adults continuing to migrate to urban areas and consequently reducing the size of potential caregivers that the disabled elderly can rely upon, the development of alternative support systems needs to be understood.

POPULATION AGING IN FIJI

Fiji consists of 330 islands, of which one third are inhabited. Located in the lower apex of the Polynesian triangle, northeast of New Zealand and bordering the International Dateline, this multi-ethnic society has benefited through primary industries in agriculture (specifically sugar), tourism, and recently, manufacturing. The elderly population in Fiji has been growing steadily over the past 30 years with the median age increasing from 16.5 to 21.2 years between 1966 and 1996. In the same period, the size of the elderly population 60 and older increased from 3.5 percent to 5.4 percent. This growth among the elderly is expected to continue, reaching 7.0 percent of the population by the year 2006 and 13.0 percent by 2026 (Fiji Bureau of Statistics, 1998; U.S. Census Bureau, 1999). The total Fiji population is almost evenly divided between ethnic Fijians and Indians whose ancestors served as indentured laborers when Fiji was under British colonial rule. In 1996, there were 39,807 individuals 60 and older of which 57 percent were Fijians and 42 percent were Indians. Elderly women outnumbered elderly men with a sex ratio of 1.06. Women also have a longer life expectancy of 69 years compared to 65 years for men (Fiji Bureau of Statistics, 1998).

Like many developing nations, care and support for the elderly in Fiji is anchored in the family. National level entitlement programs, such as social security and Medicare, are nonexistent and old age pensions are limited to only a few. Traditionally, women have cared for elderly par-

ents at home, but this type of arrangement is changing as women become educated and enter the labor force, reducing the pool of potential
caregivers. The shift to a cash based economy in Fiji has also required
women to increasingly engage in wage employment to help with family
expenses (Fiji Department for Women and Culture, 1994; Panapasa and
McNally, 1997).

Consequently, healthy and physically capable elder are increasingly
called upon to provide a series of useful functions within households in
order to compensate for declines in young female caregiver pools.
Tasks such as baby-sitting, preparing meals, and house cleaning help
offset the internal costs of care to the family and help maintain a balance
in the reciprocity calculus essential to Pacific culture (Rensel et al.,
1997; Barker, 1997). When an elderly family member becomes disabled or physically impaired, fewer of these reciprocal functions can be
performed. Simultaneously, the associated costs for medical treatment,
prescriptions and prosthetic devices for the care of the elderly can place
additional economic strains on the limited family resources. This joint
function of decreasing contribution to the family economy and increasing demands on household resources can result in stresses within the
family that adversely impact the elderly when they become impaired. A
series of studies have found the disabled elderly in Fiji to be at a higher
risk of poverty and unmet need when compared to non-disabled elderly
(Barr, 1990; Bryant, 1993; Panapasa, 2000; Plange, 1987).

DATA AND METHODOLOGY

To compare trends across time, two different data sources from two
different years are used: the 1996 Fiji Census of population and the
1995 World Health Organization (WHO) study on Health and Social
Aspects of Aging in the Western Pacific. The dependent variable is
based on a simple definition of disability on whether the elder has had
any long-term disability or health problem that negatively affects daily
activities. The independent variables are age, marital status, household
status, ethnicity, education, and residential location. These measures
have been found to be a significant predictor of disability (Lillard et al.,
1997; Kinsella et al., 1998; Plange, 1992; Briscoe, 1990).

There were 3,166 individuals age 60 and older who met the criteria
for this analysis in 1996 compared to a sample of 713 elderly respondents of the same age group for 1985. Descriptive statistics are used to
examine the characteristics of individuals with disability and to calcu-

late disability rates for each time period to provide a historical comparison of disability trends. A multivariate survival model is used to estimate the length of time before the onset of disability among elderly respondents. A multivariate logistic model is also applied to describe the risk factors that increase the likelihood of being disabled.

The theoretical discussion presented in the preceding section argues that a broad range of data and information is required to model the process of disability. Unfortunately, the realities of data content in less developed countries require that this problem be approached within the framework of a reduced model that attempts to capture the process of elderly impairment through a series of proxy variables.

ANALYSIS OF THE RESULTS

Table 1 provides a descriptive analysis of the total elderly population at risk of disability in the first column and then broken down by gender in the last two columns for Fiji in 1996. Overall, there are 37,034 elderly of which less than 10 percent experienced a disabling condition. Contrary to developed countries, disability is slightly more prevalent among men than women. Marriage remains common among the elderly with only 35 percent of the total elderly population widowed, though this is more a function of older men who remarry compared to older women where the option to remarry is limited. Overall, disability is most prevalent among older widowed women and married older men. As displayed in Table 1, the majority of older Fijians are classified as a household head or spouse. The prevalence of disability is higher among older individuals classified as a relative or parent; this is true for both older females and males. While a large proportion of older women have no education compared to older men reflecting a bias toward men, the prevalence of disability is negatively associated with increasing levels of education. As we would expect, old age disability is more prevalent in rural than urban areas where 85 percent of the elderly reside.

Figure 1 compares changes in disability rates among the elderly in 1985 and 1996. As expected, the risk of becoming disabled increased at older ages; this is true for all subgroups examined. In terms of overall rates, it appears that while the pattern of disability has remained consistent across time among women and men and subgroups examined, the onset of disability has increased at a faster rate between 1985 and 1996.

Table 2 presents a multivariate survival model that predicts the waiting time to the onset of disability by select demographic characteristics.

TABLE 1. Percent of Elderly with Disability by Select Demographic Characteristics: Fiji, 1996

	Total Population		Female Population		Male Population	
	Elderly Pop.	% Disabled	Elderly Pop.	% Disabled	Elderly Pop.	% Disabled
1996	37,034[a]	3,166	19,087	1,563	17,947	1,603
Percent	100	8.55	51.54	8.19	48.46	8.93
Age						
60-69	23,695	5.81	63.14	5.20	64.88	6.44
70-79	10,099	11.42	27.13	10.95	27.42	11.91
80+	3,240	19.63	9.73	19.87	7.71	19.31
Marital Status						
Married	23,946	7.24	47.14	5.48	83.29	8.30
Widowed	13,088	10.94	52.86	10.61	16.71	12.07
Living Arrangements						
Head/Spouse	25,150	7.62	55.51	6.51	81.10	8.42
Other Relative	11,674	10.63	43.89	10.36	18.37	11.31
Parent	7,220	11.51	28.62	11.02	9.79	13.03
Child	207	4.35	0.59	4.42	0.52	4.26
Education						
No Education	9,022	9.90	32.88	9.11	15.30	11.69
Grade School Only	18,061	8.89	46.70	8.39	50.96	9.38
Secondary or More	9,951	6.70	20.42	6.24	33.73	7.00
Ethnicity						
Fijian	21,324	9.43	57.25	9.31	57.93	9.55
Indian	15,710	7.36	42.75	6.69	42.07	8.08
Residence						
Rural	31,451	9.07	84.32	8.78	85.57	9.38
Urban	5,583	5.59	15.68	5.01	14.43	6.25

[a] *Includes Fijians and Indians only*
Source: Fiji Bureau of Statistics, 1998

FIGURE 1. Failure Rates for Disability by Age, Gender and Marital Status

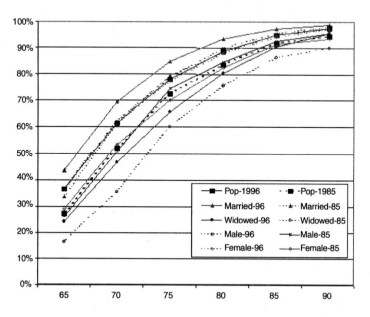

Sources: WHO Elderly Survey, 1985, and Fiji Bureau of Statistics, 1998

The first two columns represent population estimates and population odds ratios, and this sequence is then repeated for males and females. According to Table 2, the overall impacts of the control variables on the timing of disability, while highly significant, remain relatively modest. According to the overall population model, gender and urban residence represent the most powerful variable in terms of explanatory power. Women have an 11 percent slower rate of becoming disabled than men. The same is true for urban compared to rural residents. The onset of becoming disabled is 6 percent slower for Indians than Fijians with Indian females having the longest delay before becoming disabled.

As would be expected, lower levels of education are associated with an increased hazard of disability with those having a grade school education or less experiencing a decline in the timing to disability of 5 percent compared to those elderly with more than a grade school education.

TABLE 2. Multivariate Survival Model

Variable	Population Estimate	Population Odds	Males Estimate	Male Odds	Females Estimate	Female Odds
Intercept	4.8061***		4.8420***		4.8749***	
Female	0.1078***	1.1138				
Widow	−0.0127	0.9874	−0.0184	0.9817	−0.1021***	0.9030
Female & Widowed	−0.1027***	0.9024				
Indian	0.0580***	1.0597	0.0615***	1.0634	0.0977***	1.1026
Female & Indian	0.0460***	1.0470				
No Formal Education	−0.0598***	0.9419	−0.0682***	0.9341	−0.0523***	0.9491
Grade School Only	−0.0412***	0.9596	−0.0450***	0.9560	−0.0383***	0.9625
Urban Residence	0.1078***	1.1138	0.0853***	1.0890	0.1283***	1.1368
Household Head	−0.0218*	0.9784	−0.0320	0.9685	−0.0154	0.9848
Spouse of Head	−0.0732***	0.9294			−0.0582***	0.9435
Parent	−0.0590***	0.9427	−0.0629***	0.9391	−0.0557***	0.9458
Scale	0.2302	3.3433	0.2396	3.1734	0.2214	3.5163

Source: Fiji Bureau of Statistics, 1998
*$p < .05$; **$p < .01$; ***$p < .001$

Women obtain the greatest benefit from residing in urban areas gaining a 14 percent increase in the timing to disability compared to women in rural areas while men residing in urban areas gain a 9 percent increase in disability free life compared to males in rural areas.

Table 3 presents a multivariate logistic regression model of the likelihood of being disabled based on select demographic variables. Consistent with the increased risk of chronic morbidity associated with the aging life course, the likelihood of becoming disabled increases by 6 percent for each year increase in age. Overall, females are 39 percent less likely to be disabled than males, a potential outcome of cumulative differences in the roles and activities performed by men and women in Fiji and also lifestyles with drinking and smoking habits that tend to be common among men. Overall, being widowed increases the risk of being disabled by 6 percent while widowed females are 59 percent more likely to be disabled than others. When males and females are modeled independently, the gender effect of widowhood is more explicitly defined. Widowed males have a relatively low risk of disability (8 percent) compared to married males, but widowed females are 63 percent more likely to be disabled when compared to married females. These relationships are highly significant.

Consistent with the previous analysis, the logistic model finds Indians as 23 percent less likely to be disabled compared to older Fijians

TABLE 3. Multivariate Logistic Model for the Risk of Disability

Parameter	Population Estimate	Population Odds	Males Estimate	Male Odds	Females Estimate	Female Odds
Intercept	−6.8064***		−6.7112***		−7.3881***	
Age in Single Years	0.0628***	1.0648	0.0607***	1.0626	0.0650***	1.0672
Female	−0.4939***	0.6102				
Widow	0.0638	1.0659	0.0851	1.0888	0.4901***	1.6325
Female & Widowed	0.4644***	1.5911				
Indian	−0.2605***	0.7707	−0.2660***	0.7664	−0.4681***	0.6262
Female & Indian	−0.2170***	0.8049				
No Formal Education	0.2837***	1.328	0.3073***	1.3597	0.2611***	1.2984
Grade School Only	0.1945***	1.2147	0.2022***	1.2241	0.1893***	1.2084
Urban Residence	−0.4905***	0.6123	−0.3742***	0.6878	−0.6071***	0.5449
Household Head	0.1048*	1.1105	0.1448	1.1558	0.0795	1.0827
Spouse of Head	0.3404***	1.4055			0.2842***	1.3287
Parent	0.2867***	1.332	0.2915***	1.3384	0.2825***	1.3264

Source: Fiji Bureau of Statistics, 1998.
*p < .05; **p < .01; ***p < .001

with Indian females being 20 percent less likely to be disabled compared to others. Increases in the level of education have a slight insulating effect on the risk of disability regardless of gender. As expected, elderly residents in urban areas are 39 percent less likely to be disabled compared to elderly rural residents. The likelihood of being disabled increases significantly if you are the spouse or parent of the household head by over 60 percent compared to being a non-nuclear relative.

DISCUSSION AND CONCLUSIONS

This study represents an examination of the rates and patterns of disability for the elderly in Fiji. Focusing on recently released data, estimates of disability from the 1996 Census are compared with estimates derived from a 1985 World Health Organization study of the elderly in Fiji. Using lifetable techniques combined with both multivariate hazard model and logistic regression, this study identifies the speed and prevalence of disability, and its differential impacts for gender and ethnicity. The study also examines the role that disability plays in the composition of households and their location.

Implicit in the outcomes of this study is the need for more detailed data to better understand the complex relationships affecting the lives of the disabled elderly in Fiji. For example, mortality may represent an important variable in the risk of having a disabling condition. Without adequate vital statistics data it is impossible to test this assumption.

Methodologically, the data used in this analysis were limited by the approaches in which the data were collected. Unlike the detailed data on self assessed health found in the 1985 WHO survey, the census data used in this analysis is limited in the number of questions asked and the use of the household head as a proxy for the elderly respondent. A simplistic definition for disability was also adopted in the census, hence restricting the level of detail information available and providing a reduced model for analytical purposes.

Still, the data collected in the census represents valuable demographic information about the entire population, and in this case, it provides baseline information upon which detailed surveys could be developed in the future. Similarly, as census data is collected every 10 years in Fiji, repetition of these questions would allow for future comparisons.

The relationship between widowhood, gender, and disability also needs to be examined in more detail. This study show that widowed women represent a subpopulation of females at high risk of disability compared to other elderly subpopulations. Widowed females are also particularly vulnerable to poverty and unmet need for health care and support services. The pattern of selectivity towards disabled widows is also reflective of marriage market processes within Fiji. Even healthy women surviving into older ages are unlikely to remarry and the very weak may die early compared to men who often remarry after widowhood despite disabilities. Qualitative work has suggested that women who are not disabled enough to die, but disabled enough to be unattractive in the remarriage market often go on to form small independent households when they are not absorbed into the household of a child (Panapasa, 2000). These independent households are typically poor and these disabled females may receive little or no direct support from family members as their disabilities leave them unable to contribute to the large family economies that underlie Pacific exchange networks.

Another interesting finding that emerges from the study of household composition suggests that the social rank of the elderly within a household plays an important role in their ability to obtain care if disabled. While much of the policy development in Fiji regarding the elderly is based upon altruistic assumptions of traditional family support for the elderly, more recent studies have shown that the elderly who receive the best care in a household also provide high levels of services within the household. This is consistent with the reciprocal model of household economies common in Pacific societies and argues that individuals who are unable to contribute to the maintenance of the family are more likely to be abandoned or mistreated. The results from the multivariate analysis show that levels of disability within households are much lower among non-core elderly than they are for core elderly, such as the household head, spouse of head, and parents of head. This suggests that core members retain enough status and power within the household to negotiate care even with disabilities, while disabled non-core members are rare within these same households. If these disabled elderly cannot draw upon the resources of an extended household economy because they are unable to contribute to this household in a substantive way then they may be forced to maintain independent households. While not explicitly examined in this analysis, qualitative studies in Fiji have shown that such households represent seriously increased risks of poverty, unmet need, and higher rates of mortality for disabled residents (Barr, 1990; Panapasa, 2000).

With the pace of population aging in less developed countries, such as Fiji, projected to increase significantly in the future, the pace of disability and chronic impairment is expected to grow as well. With majority of the elderly residing in rural areas, the prevalence of old age disability is expected to remain high particularly in rural communities compared to urban centers. This suggests that health care systems currently offered in rural areas will need to be strengthened in anticipation of a growing future need for medical treatment and care. The living arrangement and family support system of the elderly will need to be examined in greater detail to determine the welfare of the elderly and unmet need. To face the challenges these issues and concerns imply, more detailed measures are needed to guide policy decisions in the development of programs and allocation of resources. The use of simplistic definitions for disability need to be expanded to include a more comprehensive approach as outlined earlier.

This study suggests patterns and prevalence rates of disability that will need to be addressed in the very near future. Although the pace and prevalence of disability among the elderly has grown markedly since 1985, little parallel growth has occurred in the provision of services for the elderly. This must change as the needs of the elderly will increase in the coming decades. Without substantial input from government infrastructures, families will be challenged to support the increased needs of growing numbers of older people.

While the government of Fiji is unlikely to provide direct support for the elderly, they can provide services and health care institutions for the elderly. These kinds of indirect supports allow the elderly to obtain a higher quality of life that in turn will help them maintain a productive family role. Productive contributions to the family economies increase the likelihood that they will remain within the traditional support networks that provide the direct care the government cannot duplicate. As argued in this paper, these systems are complex and heavily interdependent. Without a fuller understanding of how these interdependencies operate, it is difficult to generate rational policy.

REFERENCES

Andrews, G.R. and A.J. Esterman. 1986. *Aging in the Western Pacific*. World Health Organization Regional Office for the Western Pacific, Manila.

Barker, J. 1997. Between Humans and Ghosts: The Decrepit Elderly in Polynesian Society. In *The Cultural Context of Aging: Worldwide Perspectives*. Edited by Jay Sokolovsky. Bergin & Garvey. Westport, Connecticut.

Barr, K.J. 1990. *Poverty in Fiji. Fiji forum for justice, peace and the integrity of creation*. Suva, Fiji.

Bose, A.B. 1996. Economic and Social Conditions of the Elderly with a Special Focus on Women: Needs and Capabilities of the Elderly. In: *Implications of Asia's Population Future for Older People in the Family*. Asian Population Studies Series No. 145. United Nations, New York.

Briscoe, J. 1990. *Brazil: The new challenge of adult health*. Washington, DC: World Bank, 1990. vii, 113 p. (A World Bank Country Study).

Bryant, J.J. 1993. *Urban Poverty and the Environment in the South Pacific*. The Department of Geography and Planning, University of New England, Australia.

DaVanzo, J. and A. Chan. 1994. Living Arrangements of Older Malaysians: Who Coresides with their Adult Children? *Demography*, Volume 31, Issue 1.

Fiji Bureau of Statistics. 1998. Report on Fiji Population Census 1996: Analytical Report on the Demographic, Social and Economic Characteristics of the Population. Government Printing Office, Suva, Fiji March.

Fiji Department for Women and Culture. 1994. Women of Fiji: A Statistical Gender Profile. Government Printing Office. Suva, Fiji.

Hermalin, A.I., M. Ofstedal and M. Chang. 1996. Types of Support for the Aged and Their Providers in Taiwan. In: *Aging and Generational Relations*, Edited by Tamara K. Hareven. New York. Aldine De Gruyter.

Herzog, A.R. and R. Wallace. 1997. Measures of cognitive functioning in the AHEAD study. *Journal of Gerontology*: Series B, 52B(Special Issue) 37-48.

Kinsella, K. and Y.J. Gist. 1998. Gender and aging: Mortality and health. Washington, DC. US Census Bureau International Brief No. 98-2.

Lewis, N.D. 1998. Intellectual intersections: Gender and health in the Pacific. *Social Science & Medicine*, 46(6): 641-659.

Lillard, L. and R.J. Willis. 1997. Motives for intergenerational transfers: Evidence from Malaysia. *Demography*. February: 34(1): 115-34.

Martin, L.G. 1989a. Living arrangements of the elderly in Fiji, Korea, Malaysia and the Philippines. *Demography*, 26: 627-643.

Oliver, M. 1998. Theories in heath care research: Theories of disability in health practice and research. *British Medical Journal*, 317: 1446-1449.

Panapasa, S.V. 2000. Sociable security: Family support and elderly well-being in Fiji: 1966-1986. Unpublished doctoral dissertation for Brown University.

Panapasa, S.V. and J.W. McNally. 1997. From Cradle to Grave: Health Expectancy and Family Support Among the Elderly in Fiji. Brown University Working Paper. WP 97-10. August, 1997.

Plange, N.K. 1987. *Aspects of Ageing in Fiji.* Fiji Ageing Research, sponsored by the World Health Organization.

–1992. Attitudes, Constraints and Concerns of the Carers of the Elderly in Fiji. Unpublished survey research report. Suva, Fiji. University of the South Pacific.

Rahman, M.O. 1999. Age and gender variation in the impact of household structure on elderly mortality. *International Journal of Epidemiology*, 28: 485-491.

–1997. The impact of spouses on the mortality of older individuals in rural Bangladesh. *Health Transition Review*, 7 (1): 1-12.

Rensel, J. and A. Howard. 1997. The pace of disabled persons in Rotuman society. *Pacific Studies* 20(3): 19-50.

Smith, J.P. 1994. Measuring health and economic status of older adults in developing countries. *The Gerontologist*, 34(1): 491-496.

Smith, J. P. and R. Kington. 1997. Demographic and economic correlates of health in old age. *Demography*, 34(1): 159-170.

U.S. Bureau of the Census. 1999. Report WP/98, *World Population Profile: 1998*, U.S. Government Printing Office, Washington, DC.

Weisner, Thomas S. and Ronald Gallimore. 1977. My Brother's Keeper: Child and Sibling Caretaking. *Current Anthropology*, Vol. 18, No. 2. (Jun., 1977), pp. 169-190.

Recent Perspectives
on Active Life Expectancy
for Older Women

Sarah B. Laditka, PhD
James N. Laditka, DA, MPA

SUMMARY. This article provides a critical review of recent active life expectancy literature, describing trends of special interest to women. We review findings from leading perspectives used to study life expectancy and active life expectancy, including gender, racial and socioeconomic differences, disease-specific effects, and biodemography. We examine three competing theories of population health that frame active life expectancy research–compression of morbidity, expansion of morbidity, and dynamic equilibrium–concluding there is support for both the compression of morbidity and dynamic equilibrium theories. Policy implications for women include a greater understanding of the role of education and racial and ethnic diversity in active life trends, and an increased public pol-

Sarah B. Laditka is Associate Professor of Health Services Management, and Director, Center for Health and Aging, State University of New York Institute of Technology, P.O. Box, 3050, Utica, NY 13504 (E-mail: laditks@ sunyit.edu).

James N. Laditka is a PhD candidate at the Maxwell School of Citizenship and Public Affairs, and Research Associate of the Center for Policy Research, Syracuse University.

This research was supported, in part, by a Faculty Research Grant from the State University of New York Institute of Technology at Utica/Rome.

[Haworth co-indexing entry note]: "Recent Perspectives on Active Life Expectancy for Older Women." Laditka, Sarah B., and James N. Laditka. Co-published simultaneously in *Journal of Women & Aging* (The Haworth Press, Inc.) Vol. 14, No. 1/2, 2002, pp. 163-184; and: *Health Expectations for Older Women: International Perspectives* (ed: Sarah B. Laditka) The Haworth Press, Inc., 2002, pp. 163-184. Single or multiple copies of this article are available for a fee from The Haworth Document Delivery Service [1-800-HAWORTH 9:00 a.m. - 5:00 p.m. (EST). E-mail address: getinfo@haworthpressinc.com].

163

icy emphasis on prevention and treatment of chronic disease, together with adoption of more healthy lifestyles. *[Article copies available for a fee from The Haworth Document Delivery Service: 1-800-HAWORTH. E-mail address: <getinfo@haworthpressinc.com> Website: <http://www.HaworthPress. com> © 2002 by The Haworth Press, Inc. All rights reserved.]*

KEYWORDS. Active life expectancy, aging, longevity, healthy life expectancy, compression of morbidity, older people and health, older women, review of health trends

INTRODUCTION

Global aging will play a prominent role in shaping the 21st century (Kinsella & Gist, 1998). Many countries, both developed and developing, enjoyed dramatic life expectancy gains over the last century (U.S. Census Bureau, 2000; Vaupel et al., 1998). However, declining mortality raises new questions about life quality, especially at older ages. Do individuals who escape death from once-fatal diseases develop substantial disability from chronic diseases? Do population subgroups fare differently in life expectancy, or in the proportion of life without significant disability? Questions such as these define the study of active life expectancy, also commonly referred to as healthy life expectancy. Some researchers distinguish active life expectancy from healthy life expectancy. The latter phrase can be limited to describe only years lived without serious health problems. It is possible for an individual with health problems to remain free of serious physical or cognitive impairments when evaluated using common disability measures. It is similarly possible for a disabled individual to be free of significant health problems. Nonetheless, given the close relationship between health and physical abilities, the two phrases are often used interchangeably. Similarly, for the purposes of this review, we use the terms impairment, functional limitation, and disability interchangeably. Researchers distinguish among these terms, emphasizing that disability is in part determined by socially constructed limitations.

Policy makers and health care planners increasingly use estimates of active life expectancy to monitor changes in population health, develop health care and social policies, and forecast service costs and use. It is particularly important that women, gerontologists, and people interested in international aging understand trends in health and disability.

Women make up a large majority of most older populations (U.S. Census Bureau, 2000; Kinsella, 2000). Retirement and health policies for older persons affect women disproportionately, and these policies are driven, in part, by demographic trends. Aging populations also affect family caregiving, with important implications for both older women and their daughters. Women have dramatically increased their educational attainment, a factor that has been strongly associated both theoretically and in empirical studies of earlier generations with increasing longevity and increasing active life expectancy (Freedman & Martin, 1999; Preston, 1992). Is more education for the current generation of older women associated with longer life and a greater proportion of life spent free of disability? Or will more education simply bring more years of disability? These are particularly pressing questions addressed by recent demographic research. Individuals and their families, governments, and other social institutions all have an interest in the answers.

We present a critical review of recent active life expectancy literature. Ours is not an exhaustive review, but is intended to present general trends and leading-edge research. Our purpose is to review and critique representative theoretical articles, empirical studies, and review articles published during the past decade, with a focus on issues of special interest to women. Our spotlight is on applied work, which emphasizes findings most relevant to older individuals and their families, and to policy makers. Most methods for studying active life expectancy require accurate and detailed data about health and mortality, either for a large number of representative individuals or an entire population. Such data have generally been available only for developed countries, and the literature has largely been restricted to this focus. Although we address research on less developed countries, our review is for the most part similarly bounded. We begin, in the following section, by summarizing the most important approaches to the study of both total and active life expectancy. Here, we also describe major findings of recent empirical studies conducted using each approach. We then discuss several competing theories of population health that frame the active life expectancy literature. These theories are commonly referred to as the "compression of morbidity," the "expansion of morbidity," and "dynamic equilibrium." Briefly, the compression of morbidity theory suggests that people are living a greater proportion of life free of disease and disability. In contrast, proponents of the expansion of morbidity suggest that the percentage of life lived with disability is growing. Dynamic equilibrium offers the view that the disabled proportion of the population will increase as mortality rates fall, but that this increase will be accompanied by a reduction in the rate at which chronic diseases progress. We review active life expectancy findings from the perspective of each theory. Finally, we discuss policy implications of these collective findings, with particular emphasis on implications for women.

LEADING PERSPECTIVES AND FINDINGS

Gender Differences

Almost all studies have found that life expectancy is notably longer for women than for men, but that women spend a greater proportion of their longer lives with significant disability (Robine, Romieu, & Cambois, 1997). This is the case for women living in European countries such as France, The Netherlands, England, and Wales, as well as Canada (Bélanger, Martel, Berthelot, & Wilkins, 2002; Robine & Ritchie, 1991) and Japan (Sauvaget, Tsuji, Aonuma, & Hisamichi, 1999; Tsuji, Sauvaget, & Hisamichi, 2002). This has also been the finding of numerous studies conducted using data from the United States (e.g., Branch et al., 1991; Crimmins, Hayward, & Saito, 1996; Laditka & Wolf, 1998; Manton, Corder, & Stallard, 1993). Recent findings highlight gender differences in developing and developed counties throughout the world as well as in relatively homogeneous European countries (Mathers, Murray, Lopez, Sadana, & Salomon, 2002; Robine, Jagger, & Cambois, 2002). Several reasons are cited for these substantial gender differences in life expectancy and active life expectancy. Some researchers find that women have more favorable survival histories than men at all ages. Thus, women's advantage at later ages merely continues trends of earlier life stages (Deeg, 2001). Women are more likely to experience a decline in functional status, and are less likely to recover than men (Becket et al., 1996). Others conclude that the somewhat higher incidence of disability among women *at all ages* accounts for substantial gender differences in disability prevalence at older ages (Leveille, Penninx, Melzer, Izmirlian, & Guralnik, 2000). Women may simply accumulate more disability throughout the life course.

Socioeconomic Differences

Researchers calculating active life expectancy have often used two broad measures to capture differences in socioeconomic status, income, and education. For the measure of income, reviewing studies using data from Canada, The Netherlands, Finland and Belgium, Bone, Bebbington, and Nicolaas (1998), and Robine and Ritchie (1991) conclude that more affluent people live substantially longer and healthier lives than the less affluent. These income differences in life expectancy and active life expectancy are greater than gender differences. Education has a similar relationship to health. It seems clear, at least from studies using United States' data, that older women and men with more education live longer, healthier lives than people with less education (Crimmins et al., 1996; Crimmins & Saito, 2001; Freedman & Martin, 1999; Laditka & Wolf, 1998; Land, Guralnik, & Blazer, 1994). Using data from Fiji, Panapasa (2002) also found that more education was positively associated with longer, healthier lives for women and men. Researchers have suggested several ways that education may confer protective effects relating to specific functional limitations and major diseases. Education may alter one's ability to understand risks to health, or the propensity to accept or reduce known risks. For example, taking vitamin supplements and not smoking may protect against macular degeneration and cataracts, and thereby reduce visual impairment at older ages (e.g., Christen, Glynn, & Hennekens, 1996). Increased physical activity, improved diet, and weight control have also been linked to more education. These lifestyle advantages are further linked to reduced levels of some chronic conditions, such as arthritis and osteoporosis (Wister, 1996). There is evidence that women with less education have substantially more behavioral and biological risks associated with coronary artery disease. For example, they are more likely to smoke cigarettes, exercise less, and have lower high-density lipoprotein levels than women with more education (Matthews, Kelsey, Meilahn, Kuller, & Wing, 1989). When both income and education are included in the research design, women and men living in Belgium, Canada, Finland, The Netherlands, and Sweden who are poorer and have less education live shorter, more disabled lives than those who are more affluent and have more education (Robine et al., 1997).

Racial Differences

Most studies of racial differences in active life expectancy have been restricted to data from the United States, most often comparing active life expectancies of whites and blacks. These life expectancy comparisons invariably report that death rates for blacks exceed those of whites at younger ages. In some studies, curves plotting life expectancy at each age for blacks and whites cross at older ages (80 and over). In these studies, death rate estimates for whites exceed those for blacks at these older ages. Demographers intensely debate the existence of a black-white mortality crossover. Some argue that any evidence of a crossover reflects inaccurate age reporting by older people. Several studies have corrected for age misstatement by survey respondents. In these studies, the black-white crossover disappeared (Elo & Preston, 1997; Preston, Elo, Rosenwaike, & Hill, 1996). Manton and Stallard (1997), however, found evidence of a mortality crossover even after correcting for age misstatement. They found that, among those having reached old age, blacks live longer, more disabled lives than whites. Consistent with gender differences for whites, researchers generally find that black women live substantially longer than black men. In a study that corrected for age misstatement and examined longevity trends from the late 1930s until 1990, Elo (2001) found life expectancy gains of almost 20 years for black women and 14 years for black men. During the latter half of the twentieth century, Elo found black women achieved notably larger gains in life expectancy than black men.

There is also evidence of morbidity differences between blacks and whites. Several researchers have found that, compared with whites, blacks at older ages are less likely to be disabled, and have longer life expectancies. For example, Clark, Maddox, and Steinhauser (1993) found that blacks age 85 or older are only about 50% as likely to experience a decline in functional status as whites. Land et al. (1994) found that black women and men age 75 or older had both active and impaired life expectancies noticeably exceeding those of white women and men. However, a growing number of researchers have found that white women and men have both total and active life expectancies longer than those of black women and men (Crimmins et al., 1996; Geronimus, Bound, Waidmann, Colen, & Steffick, 2001; Hayward & Heron, 1999). In addition, most researchers conclude that black women live a notably greater percentage of their lives with disability than black men (e.g., Crimmins et al., 1996; Crimmins & Saito, 2001; Geronimus et al., 2001; Hayward & Heron, 1999). A small number of studies have examined life expectancy and disability patterns for other racial and ethnic groups. These studies have found that blacks and native Americans live notably shorter and more disabled lives than whites, Asian Americans, or Hispanics (Hayward & Heron, 1999; Waidmann & Liu, 2000). Researchers emphasize disparate distributions of advantages and disadvantages over the life span, and socioeconomic and cultural factors as likely causes of racial and ethnic disparities in mortality and morbidity

(Blackwell, Hayward, & Crimmins, 2001; Hayward, Crimmins, Miles, & Yang, 2000).

Additional Health Status Indicators

Health encompasses multiple dimensions. Researchers therefore stress the importance of incorporating multiple dimensions of health in studies examining life expectancy and active life expectancy (Crimmins, 1996). Panapasa (2002) describes the complexity of defining disability in developing countries, where disability is influenced by factors beyond those generally found in social and medical support systems of developed countries. Many studies have used one or both of two standard measures to represent functional status: Activities of Daily Living (ADLs) such as eating, dressing, and bathing, and Instrumental Activities of Daily Living (IADLs) such as marketing and preparing meals (Branch et al., 1991; Crimmins, Hayward, & Saito, 1994, 1996; Laditka & Wolf, 1998; Manton, Corder, & Stallard, 1993; Manton & Gu, 2001). Wolf, Laditka, and Laditka (2002) provide a new perspective on ADL disability by reporting the full distribution of remaining total, active, and inactive years for women sharing a set of important characteristics. Wolf et al. (2002) found that years of total, active, and inactive life are broadly distributed within each group of women with the same characteristics. They also found that the shapes of these distributions vary considerably across groups, highlighting the heterogeneity of disability in older populations.

Recently, sensory and cognitive impairments have been added to the set of functional status measures included in definitions of active and impaired life. Jagger, Raymond, and Morgan (1998) found that women live a greater proportion of life with impaired vision than men. Vision impairment is a particularly interesting indicator of functional status when the research focus is on changing disability patterns. Treatments for vision impairments have improved markedly in recent years, as exemplified by treatments for cataracts and diabetic retinopathy. These improvements are likely to have substantial positive effects on the ability of older people to live independently. Jagger and Matthews (2002) included cognitive status as a disability measure, and found that women live a substantially longer proportion of remaining life with a cognitive impairment than men. Cognitive deterioration is of increasing interest, because extended longevity has been accompanied by predictions of more dementia, especially for women (e.g., Brookmeyer, Gray, & Kawas, 1998).

Some researchers suggest that ADLs and IADLs are strongly influenced by individuals' socially defined roles and physical environments. An individual may be less likely to report disability if she can compensate for an impairment with assistive devices, or by upgrading her home to aid functioning. A woman who might otherwise be disabled in bathing by some measures, for example, might regain her ability to perform this activity with a walk-in shower or tub. Changes in functioning found by recent research could reflect changes in individuals' expectations of disability and use of equipment, rather than changes in their underlying physiological functioning (Crimmins, 1996; Freedman & Martin, 1998). An increasing number of studies have used measures such as seeing, lifting, carrying, and climbing stairs, instead of–or in addition to–ADL and/or IADL scales, to capture more information about underlying physiological functioning (Freedman & Martin, 1998, 1999, 2000; Jagger et al., 1998; Leveille et al., 2000; Waidmann & Liu, 2000). In another area, studies have also used self-reported health, often in conjunction with other health indicators (Spiers, Jagger, & Clarke, 1996). However, there is evidence of gender differences in the ways in which women and men evaluate and report their own health status. For example, Helmer, Barberger-Gateau, Letenneur, and Dartigues (1999) found that self-reported health was more closely associated with medical conditions and disability for women than for men. Thus, the predictive power of subjective health reports from women and men may differ.

"Health profiles" identified with the Grade of Membership (GoM) method offer another measure of health status for active life expectancy research. This method groups individuals based on the types and extent of health problems they experience (Manton, Woodbury, Stallard, & Corder, 1992). The GoM method often incorporates information about co-morbidity as well as degree of disability. Deeg, Portrait, and Lindeboom (2002) identified six health profiles for women and men in The Netherlands. They found that women are more likely than men to be frail, to have cancer, or to be cognitively impaired.

Disease Specific Effects

An additional dimension of disability is captured by examining cause-specific mortality and/or morbidity rates, and their effects on active life expectancy. Research in this area is often restricted by the limited availability of sufficiently detailed data. For example, analyses generally do not account for co-morbidities, which could provide a measure of underlying health status, and other risk factors. Where appropriate data are available, however, this approach allows researchers to rank diseases by their importance in contributing to mortality and morbidity. Findings in this area are particularly useful for policy makers, because they provide information that can be used to select among alternative strategies targeted toward specific diseases. By quantifying hypothetical gains to total life and active life, these methods provide a basis for ranking research funding options for acute and chronic diseases.

Cause-specific mortality and morbidity calculations have been made using data from Australia, Canada, The Netherlands, the United Kingdom, and the United States (Bélanger et al., 2002; Robine et al., 1997). Reviewing results from Australia, Britain, and The Netherlands, and focusing on three major disease categories–cancer, circulatory disease, and musculoskeletal conditions–Bone et al. (1998) found that eliminating circulatory diseases had the largest positive effect on longevity. Eliminating chronic nonfatal diseases, such as musculoskeletal conditions, had almost no effect on life expectancy, but brought the largest gain in the proportion of active life for most people studied (Bone et al., 1998; Nusselder, van der Velden, van Sonsbeek, Lenior, & van den Bos, 1996). Estimating models in which a major cause of death was eliminated separately for women and men, Hayward, Crimmins, and Saito (1998) found substantial gender differences in disease-specific effects. For both women and men, eliminating heart disease brought the greatest life expectancy gains. For men, additional years from the elimination of heart disease were primarily active ones (Hayward et al., 1998). For women, however, these years gained were inactive years. Providing another perspective on disease-specific effects, Crimmins, Kim, and Hagedorn (2002) compared life with and without major diseases between women and men. They found that women live longer with and without diseases than men. Interestingly, they found that women live longer with heart disease than men, despite notably later disease onset. They also found that men live longer with arthritis than they do with heart disease.

Biodemography

Biodemography is one of the most recent approaches to active life expectancy. Biodemography integrates demographic methods with applications from the biological sciences, and examines the role of biological factors in life expectancy. Biodemography allows researchers to address questions about the influence of genes and the environment on the course of aging and survival. Biodemography addresses questions about the nature of processes that underlie demographic trends, and population aging and health. How might genetic components of differential aging rates affect gender differences in mortality? What are the reasons for observed mortality decline? How long will this trend continue? What are the biological limits of human longevity? Why do some individuals die shortly after birth, while others live to old age? Questions such as these stimulate new approaches to longstanding demographic mysteries, such the gender gap in longevity. Wachter (1997) provides a useful review of biodemography perspectives, stressing that, in contrast to focusing on limits to life expectancy and built-in senescence, more recent views emphasize the plasticity of the life span.

Two empirical studies illustrate recent analyses in biodemography, and highlight research important for women. Using historical data for European aristocratic families, Gavrilov and Gavrilova (2001) examined health and longevity trends for daughters and sons born to parents of various ages. Their unusual study population offered the distinct advantage of relatively uniform lifestyles, and thus implicitly controlled for many factors that otherwise challenge the interpretability of demographic research. Their primary question was: Does parental age affect health and longevity differently for daughters and sons? They found that parental age influences the life span for daughters but not for sons: daughters born to older fathers (45 to 55 years) had significantly shorter lives than daughters born to younger fathers. The age of the mother was not significantly associated with longevity for daughters or sons. Reasoning from the perspective of biodemography, Gavrilov and Gavrilova observe that only daughters inherit the paternal X chromosome. Given their findings, they speculate that the X chromosome may concentrate genes that affect longevity and are sensitive to mutation. If confirmed by further research, this finding would have important implications for women, because there has been a dramatic increase in childbearing at older ages in many countries.

In another study examining the degree to which daughters and sons might inherit genes that affect their life spans, Cournil (2001) used data from a historical population registry, analyzing people from a small homogeneous rural farming community. Since members of this community shared similar lifestyles and education levels, wealth, and so forth, the population choice controlled for socioeconomic status and lifestyle. Sons' longevity was not influenced by their mothers' or fathers' length of life. Mothers' longevity was also not significantly related to either daughters' or sons' longevity. But Cournil found that daughters of short-lived fathers had notably shorter life spans than daughters of longer lived fathers. Similar to Gavrilov and Gavrilova (2001), Cournil suggests that this result indicates an important role for the X chromosome in women's longevity.

MORBIDITY COMPRESSION, EXPANSION, OR DYNAMIC EQUILIBRIUM?

The active life expectancy literature is framed by three competing theories of trends in population health. Fries (1980) proposed that the onset of illness and disability could be postponed to a brief period at the end of life. Fries' theory is often referred to as the compression of morbidity. In contrast, representing the expansion of morbidity theory, Gruenberg (1977) and Kramer (1983) argued that longer lives will be accompanied by more chronic disease and disability. The theory of dynamic equilibrium, proposed by Manton (1982), assumes a more complex dynamic for population health. As mortality rates fall, it suggests, the prevalence of chronic disease will increase. At the same time, the rate at which chronic diseases progress will slow. In sum, more people will be disabled, and they will be disabled through more years. But through many of this increased number of years, they will experience less intense forms of disability. When examining evidence for these theories, researchers have studied trends in both incidence and prevalence. Incidence refers to the onset of new cases of health problems, such as disability or disease. Prevalence refers to the percentage of the population experiencing the disease or disability at a given time. We describe approaches used to address these theories, review findings of empirical work, and consider how these findings tend to support or refute the three theories.

Observed Changes in Population Health

Research using data from the 1960s and 1970s found that older Americans were then living longer, but in poorer health (Colvez & Blanchet, 1981; Crimmins, Saito, & Ingegneri, 1989; Verbrugge, 1984). More recently, most studies from the early 1980s to the late 1990s indicate improving health for older women and men. Using data from the National Long-Term Care Survey (NLTCS), Manton and colleagues found that the prevalence of disability decreased from the early 1980s to the late 1980s (Manton, Corder, & Stallard, 1993). Another study found evidence of both increased life expectancy and small increases in healthy life expectancy (Crimmins, Saito, & Ingegneri, 1997). One study found no clear trends in disability prevalence (Crimmins, Saito, & Reynolds, 1997). Reviewing evidence from the 1982 to 1989 NLTCS and 1984 to 1990 Longitudinal Study of Aging, Freedman and Soldo (1994) concluded there was evidence of reductions in the prevalence of IADL disability and in the incidence of ADL and IADL disability.

Studies using more recent data have also found significant disability declines. Using data from 1982 to 1994 and adjusting for age, Manton, Corder, and Stallard (1997) found there was a 1.1% annual relative decline in the proportion of people who were chronically disabled (having an ADL disability that had lasted, or that was expected to last, 90 or more days at the time of interview). Using different functional status measures, Freedman and Martin (1998) analyzed data from 1983 and 1994, also finding significant limitation reductions. These reductions amounted to 0.9% to 2.3% annually, depending on the measure of functional status examined. The biggest limitation reductions were among the oldest old, people age 80 or over, suggesting the plasticity of age-related diseases even at older ages. Using data from 1983 to 1993 and four measures of functional ability (seeing, lifting and carrying, climbing stairs, and walking a quarter mile), Freedman and Martin (1999) found significant reductions in all measures of functional limitation. They also found that increased educational attainment for the cohort reaching older ages during this period accounted for the largest share of the improvement. Waidmann and Liu (2000) used Medicare Current Beneficiary Survey data from 1992 to 1996, and found that the largest decreases were in IADL disability, reductions of 2.3% per year, after controlling for age and sex. Studying trends from 1978 through 1998 for the Austrian population, Doblhammer and Kytir (2001) found the proportion of life lived in good health increased throughout the period for women and men, and that mortality rates declined throughout the period. Examining trends in several U.S. studies, Schoeni, Freedman, and Wallace (2001) conclude that improvements in health were concentrated in the 1982 to 1986 period, and more modest declines were evident from 1992 through 1996. Decreases in disability during these periods occurred for women and men, and were concentrated in individuals with higher education (Schoeni et al., 2001). Using data from the NLTCS that included surveys from 1982 through 1999, Manton and Gu (2001) reach a different conclusion. They found that the rate of decrease in the prevalence of chronic disability was greater in the 1990s than the 1980s; the standardized annual rate of decrease in the prevalence of disability was 0.26% from 1982 to 1989, 0.38% from 1989 to 1994, and 0.56% from 1994 to 1999 (Manton & Gu, 2001). These researchers also found that blacks experienced a larger percentage decline in disability prevalence than nonblacks (Manton & Gu, 2001). Collectively, these studies offer support for the compression of morbidity theory, and suggest that the older population was healthier in the 1980s and 1990s than it was in the 1960s and 1970s.

Two recent studies focus on links between disability prevalence and reports of major chronic diseases. Using data from 1981 and 1991 in France, Robine, Mormiche, and Sermet (1998) found a notable decrease in the prevalence of disability among middle aged and older people. However, they also found that the prevalence of thirteen major chronic diseases (e.g., cancer, heart disease) increased during this period. They suggest that the most frequent chronic diseases, cardiovascular disease and arthritis, appear to be less disabling in 1991 than in 1981. Freedman and Martin (2000) also examined the link between chronic disease and functioning, using samples of older Americans from 1984 and 1994. They developed two scales of functional status: one for upper body limitation, one for lower body limitation. They also examined prevalence for nine major chronic diseases and injuries (e.g., hip fracture, cancer, heart disease, and arthritis). Lower body limitations declined significantly, about 1.4% annually. If disability reductions of this magnitude were to continue over an extended period, the change would alter the face of aging importantly, both for individuals and their families, and in terms of costs to the nation. Despite declining functional limitations, however, reports of all chronic diseases and injuries increased in the Freedman and Martin study, with the exception of hypertension. Similar to Robine et al. (1998), Freedman and Martin (2000) found that several major diseases, particularly arthritis, appeared to be less debilitating for more recent cohorts of older individuals. These researchers suggest their findings may arise from earlier disease detection, advances in treatment, and reductions in behavioral risks, such as poor diet or lack of exercise. These two studies offer support for the dynamic equilibrium theory.

Also supporting the theory of dynamic equilibrium is a study by Spiers et al. (1996), who used 1981 and 1988 data from the United Kingdom to examine trends in both functional status, measured by ADLs, and self-reported health. They found a significant reduction in the proportion of older people who were dependent in at least one of five

ADLs. However, respondents surveyed in 1988 were less likely to report good health than those surveyed in 1981. This seemingly contradictory finding of improved ADL functioning and reduced self perceived health status underscores the multidimensional nature of population health, and highlights the importance of including disability measures spanning severe and mild impairments. It also has important policy implications. As Spiers et al. (1996) emphasize, the way people perceive their own health status may be influenced by both the absolute and relative prevalence of severe and mild chronic conditions in their society. In the scenario painted by their research findings, the population makes headway against severe disability while experiencing more mild disability. Here, the threshold at which individuals perceive "disability" may be lowered for everyone. As individuals approach that lowered threshold, they may seek treatment or other services for conditions or impairment levels that would not have prompted concern for many individuals of earlier cohorts. To the extent that heightened expectations spur improved medical management, technological developments, and healthier lifestyles, they may lead to further improvements in population health. However, these improvements may entail increased costs. Paradoxically, these improvements can also increase reported rates of disability.

Demographic Models of Population Health

Scholars have also used data from a number of countries, and various demographic methods, to simulate effects of mortality and/or morbidity changes on life expectancy and active life expectancy. Reviewing findings in this area, Bone et al. (1998) conclude that the most likely way we might bring about morbidity compression would be to delay the onset of chronic disease, increase remission rates, and focus on chronic diseases that seldom cause death but produce a large proportion of morbidity and disability. Crimmins et al. (1994) illustrate separate and combined effects of changing assumptions about mortality and morbidity. Crimmins and her colleagues conclude that increasing the age at which individuals become disabled or decreasing the incidence of disability are the most effective ways to reduce the number of people with a functional limitation. Do various population subgroups fare differently with generally improving health? Laditka and Laditka (2001) addressed this question by examining effects of reducing morbidity on expectancies for total and active life for several subgroups of older individuals. Women experienced greater proportional gains in both total and active life expectancy than men in their simulations. Nonwhites experienced larger proportional gains in both total and active life expectancy than whites. Women and men with less education had greater proportional gains in both total and active life expectancy than those with more education. Thus, women and traditionally disadvantaged population subgroups had the most to gain, in terms of active life expectancy, by reducing functional decline and increasing recovery from illness or injury.

Several simulation studies have explicitly modeled effects of improved education. Waidmann and Liu (2000) estimated projections of older people through 2040 under several scenarios. For the baseline projection, they assumed the current prevalence of disability stayed constant. When they assumed that improvements observed between 1992 and 1996 continue to accumulate at the same rate indefinitely, there was about a 62% reduction in IADL disability and a 50% decrease in ADL disability. In addition, Waidmann and Liu suggest that we already may have achieved most of the gains in functional status obtainable from more education. Using data from 1984 to 1993 and a different modeling approach, Freedman and Martin (1999) reach a similar conclusion about smaller disability improvements attributed to future gains in education. Freedman and Martin (1999) project functional status through 2030 under several assumptions of changes in education, holding all other factors constant. Over the period of their projection, changes in education decreased functional difficulty by 1.3% to 3.2%, depending on the disability measure selected. These researchers suggest that future disability reductions will be small, compared with improvements of the recent past.

CONCLUSIONS AND POLICY IMPLICATIONS

Our review of the active life expectancy literature suggests several important policy implications. Socioeconomic factors, particularly education, are significantly associated with expectancies for longevity and active life. Results from several recent studies suggest that most of the benefits attributed to more education have already been achieved. But there may be differential effects of education for women. Women coming of age in recent decades have achieved greater educational gains than men. In developing countries, women are still often disadvantaged in educational opportunity; yet here, too, women are beginning to experience relative education gains.

Better data and emerging methodologies will continue to improve our understanding of longevity and the dynamics of population health. Further research is particularly likely to shed light on trends in population health and inform policy making in three areas: total and active life differences for at-risk populations such as those defined by race, ethnicity, or income, active life expectancy estimates for developing countries, and biodemography. Based on current trends, by the year 2025 over two thirds of older women will live in developing countries (Kinsella & Gist, 1998). Thus, a better understanding of population health trends in developing countries, where population growth is great and resources are much harder to come by, is important (Panapasa, 2002). Biodemography is another area in which more research is needed. Biodemography has already shed new light on possible reasons for longevity differences between women and men. Future work in this area will likely help us better understand processes underlying active life expectancy differences, too. Advances in genetics, like mapping the human genome, should spur this work. Biodemographers can now expect to learn more about causal impacts of specific genes on medical conditions involved in longevity and active life.

Also useful for setting policy priorities is information about relative effects of various lethal and chronic diseases on longevity and active life expectancy. Results from cause-specific studies of major diseases suggest that eliminating lethal diseases, such as heart disease, increases the proportion of disabled life for women. Eliminating nonfatal disabling diseases, such as arthritis and osteoporosis, increases the percentage of active life, and thereby quality of life. A substantially higher percentage of women than men suffer from chronic diseases, so women have a special interest in policies that help find ways to prevent, delay, or treat nonfatal or chronic diseases.

Findings for the three theories of population health, compression of morbidity, expansion of morbidity, and dynamic equilibrium, are complex–and remain inconclusive. A growing number of studies offer evidence of improving population health over the past decade, supporting the compression of morbidity theory (e.g., Freedman & Martin, 1998; Manton et al., 1997; Manton & Gu, 2001). Collectively, however, studies in this area also tend to support the theory of dynamic equilibrium described by Manton (1982) (Crimmins, Saito, & Reynolds, 1997; Freedman & Martin, 2000; Robine et al., 1998; Spiers et al., 1996).

Despite mixed findings about population health trends, two results of active life expectancy research are clear. First, women are more likely than men to become disabled. When women experience disability, they are also less likely to recover. Thus, women have higher disability incidence and prevalence at all ages (e.g., Becket et al., 1996; Leveille et al., 2000). Second, studies using demographic models to examine population health demonstrate that the greatest gains in longevity and active life expectancy come by decreasing the rate of functional status decline (e.g., Crimmins et al., 1994; Laditka & Laditka, 2001). Regardless of which of the three competing theories of population health might come closest to actual population processes in the coming decades, many researchers familiar with these issues agree that more public resources should be devoted to preventing or delaying the onset of disabling diseases (e.g., Crimmins, Saito, & Reynolds, 1997; Laditka & Laditka, 2000, 2001).

This view is supported by a growing body of research that shows women and men who adopt healthy lifestyles–controlling blood pressure, maintaining appropriate weight, abstaining from smoking, and being physically active–have a significantly lower prevalence of illness and impairment than those who do not follow healthy lifestyles (e.g., Reed et al., 1998; Vita Terry, Hubert, & Fries, 1998). These findings suggest that policy makers and practitioners serving older people should become more proactive in promoting exercise and generally healthier lifestyles. Enhancing public investment in healthy lifestyles will reward women disproportionately, given their longer lives, their greater incidence of both chronic illness and disability, and their greater use of long-term care. If healthy lifestyles are associated with morbidity compression and their adoption is promoted successfully, women's long-term care needs would be substantially reduced. The care women commonly provide for their parents and husbands would be reduced as well.

Research on disability processes often overlooks the fact that the great majority of individuals at all but the very oldest ages live relatively active lives. They may have minor impairments that limit one activity or another, and these limitations can eventually become sufficiently restrictive that life becomes inactive, disabled, by common health status measures. Even an individual living a joyous, productive, and otherwise active life might find herself responding "yes" to the phrasing of a survey question asking about a particular impairment. The reality of life for us all is that the distinction between "active" life and "inactive" life disguises a continuum of functional ability. Recognizing this continuum only adds to the complexity of active life expectancy research, already illustrated in our review.

Regardless of the thresholds we may set defining disability, however, long-term care will exert pressing demands on our society's resources in the coming decades. We face these increasing pressures no matter what actions we may take to ameliorate the impact of population aging. The large baby boom cohort will require more formal and informal care, in the aggregate, regardless of lifestyle changes, or research successes, or morbidity compression we may enjoy. Nonetheless, our review suggests, as nations and individuals, we can still do more to limit decline, enhance recovery, and extend active life.

REFERENCES

Becket, L.A., Brock, D.B., Lemke, J.H., Mendes de Leon, C. Guralnik, J.M., Fillenbaum, G.G., Branch, L.G., Wetle, T.T., & Evans, D.A. (1996). Analysis of change in self-reported physical function among older persons in four population studies. *American Journal of Epidemiology, 143*, 766-778.

Bélanger, A., Martel, L., Berthelot, J.M., & Wilkins, R. (2002). Gender differences in disability-free life expectancy for selected risk factors and chronic conditions in Canada. *Journal of Women & Aging, 14*, 168.

Blackwell, D.L., Hayward, M.D., & Crimmins, E.M. (2001). Does childhood health affect chronic morbidity in later life? *Social Science & Medicine, 52*, 1269-1284.

Bone, M.R., Bebbington, A.C., & Nicolaas, G. (1998). Policy applications of health expectancy. *Journal of Aging and Health, 10*, 136-153.

Branch, L.G., Guralnik, J.M., Foley, D.J., Kohout, F.J., Wetle, T.T., Ostfeld, A., & Katz, S. (1991). Active life expectancy for 10,000 Caucasian men and women in three communities. *Journal of Gerontology: Medical Sciences, 46*, M145-M150.

Brookmeyer, R., Gray, S., & Kawas, C. (1998). Projections of Alzheimer's disease in the United States and the public health impact of delaying disease onset. *American Journal of Public Health, 88*, 1337-1342.

Christen, W.G., Glynn, R.J., & Hennekens, C.H. (1996). Antioxidants and age-related eye disease. *Annuls of Epidemiology, 6*, 60-66.

Clark, D.O., Maddox, G.L., & Steinhauser, K. (1993). Race, aging, and functional health. *Journal of Aging and Health, 5*, 536-553.

Colvez, A., & Blanchet, M. (1981). Disability trends in the United States population 1966-76: Analysis of reported causes. *American Journal of Public Health, 71*, 464-471.

Cournil, A. (2001). Gender-linked effects on the inheritance of longevity, a population-based study: Valserine Valley XVIII-XXth. In J.M. Robine, T.B.L. Kirkwood, & M. Allard (Eds.), *Sex and longevity: Sexuality, gender, reproduction, parenthood* (pp. 33-42). New York: Springer-Verlag.

Crimmins, E.M. (1996). Mixed trends in population health among older adults. *Journal of Gerontology: Social Sciences, 51B*, S223-S225.

Crimmins, E.M., Hayward, M.D., & Saito, Y. (1994). Changing mortality and morbidity rates and the health status and life expectancy of the older population. *Demography, 31*, 159-175.

Crimmins, E.M., Hayward, M.D., & Saito, Y. (1996). Differentials in active life expectancy in the older population of the United States. *Journal of Gerontology: Social Sciences, 51B*, S111-S120.

Crimmins, E.M., Kim, J.K., & Hagedorn, A. (2002). Life with and without disease: Women experience more of both. *Journal of Women & Aging, 14*, 173.

Crimmins, E.M., & Saito,Y. (2001). Trends in healthy life expectancy in the United States, 1970-1999: Gender, racial, and educational differences. *Social Science & Medicine, 52*, 1629-1641.

Crimmins, E.M., Saito,Y., & Ingegneri, D. (1989). Changes in life expectancy and disability-free life expectancy in the United States. *Population and Development Review, 15*, 235-267.

Crimmins, E.M., Saito,Y., & Ingegneri, D. (1997). Trends in disability-free life expectancy in the United States, 1970-90. *Population and Development Review, 23*, 555-572.

Crimmins, E.M., Saito, Y., & Reynolds, S.L. (1997). Further evidence on recent trends in the prevalence and incidence of disability among older Americans from two sources: The LSOA and the NHIS. *Journal of Gerontology: Social Sciences, 52B*, S59-S71.

Deeg, D.J.H. (2001). Sex-differences in the evolution of life expectancy and health in old age. In J.M. Robine, T.B.L. Kirkwood, & M. Allard (Eds.), *Sex and longevity: Sexuality, gender, reproduction, parenthood* (pp. 129-140). New York: Springer-Verlag.

Deeg, D.J.H., Portrait, F., & Lindeboom, M. (2002). Health profiles and profile-specific health expectancies of older women and men: The Netherlands. *Journal of Women & Aging, 14*, 172.

Doblhammer, G., & Kytir, J. (2001). Compression or expansion of morbidity? Trends in healthy-life expectancy in the elderly Austrian population between 1978 and 1998. *Social Science & Medicine, 52*, 385-391.

Elo, I.T. (2001). New African American life tables from 1935-1940 to 1985-1990. *Demography, 38*, 97-114.

Elo, I.T., & Preston, S.H. (1997). Racial and ethnic differences in mortality at older ages. In L.G. Martin & B.J. Soldo (Eds.), *Racial and ethnic differences in the health of older Americans* (pp. 10-42). Washington, DC: National Academy Press.

Freedman, V.A., & Martin, L.G. (2000). Contributions of chronic conditions to aggregate changes in old-age functioning. *American Journal of Public Health, 90*, 1755-1760.

Freedman, V.A., & Martin, L.G. (1999). The role of education in explaining and forecasting trends in functional limitations among older Americans. *Demography, 36*, 461-473.

Freedman, V.A., & Martin, L.G. (1998). Understanding trends in functional limitations among older Americans. *American Journal of Public Health, 88*, 1457-1462.

Freedman, V.A., & Soldo, B.J. (Eds.) (1994). *Trends in disability at older ages: Summary of a workshop*. Washington, DC: National Academy Press.

Fries, J.F. (1980). Aging, natural death, and the compression of morbidity. *New England Journal of Medicine, 303*, 130-135.

Gavrilov, L.A., & Gavrilova, N.S. (2001). Human longevity and parental age at conception. In J.M. Robine, T.B.L. Kirkwood, & M. Allard (Eds.), *Sex and longevity: Sexuality, gender, reproduction, parenthood* (pp. 7-31). New York: Springer-Verlag.

Geronimus, A.T., Bound, J., Waidmann, T.A., Colen, C.G., & Steffick, D. (2001). Inequity in life expectancy, functional status, and active life expectancy across selected black and white populations in the United States. *Demography, 38*, 227-251.

Gruenberg, E.M. (1977). The failures of success. *Milbank Memorial Fund Quarterly, 55*, 3-24.

Hayward, M.D., Crimmins, E.M., Miles, T.P., & Yang, Y. (2000). The significance of socioeconomic status in explaining the racial gap in chronic health conditions. *American Sociological Review, 65*, 910-930.

Hayward, M.D., Crimmins, E.M. & Saito, Y. (1998). Causes of death and active life expectancy in the older population of the United States. *Journal of Aging and Health, 10*, 192-213.

Hayward, M.D., & Heron, M. (1999). Racial inequity in active life among adult Americans. *Demography, 36*, 77-91.

Helmer, C., Barberger-Gateau, P., Letenneur, L., & Dartigues, J.F. (1999). Subjective health and mortality in French elderly women and men. *Journal of Gerontology: Social Sciences, 54B*, S84-S92.

Jagger, C., & Matthews, F. (2002). Gender differences in life expectancy free of impairment at older ages. *Journal of Women & Aging, 14*, 171.

Jagger, C., Raymond, N., & Morgan, K. (1998). Planning for the future: The effect of changing mortality, incidence, and recovery rates on life expectancy with visual disability. *Journal of Aging and Health, 10*, 154-170.

Kinsella, K. (2000). Demographic dimensions of global aging. *Journal of Family Issues, 21*, 542-558.

Kinsella, K., & Gist, Y.J. (1998). *International brief: Gender and aging*. Washington, DC: Bureau of the Census.

Kramer, M. (1983). The increasing prevalence of mental disorders: A pandemic threat. *Psychiatric Quarterly, 55*, 115-143.

Laditka, J.N., & Laditka, S.B. (2000). The morbidity compression debate: Risks, opportunities, and policy options for women. *Journal of Women & Aging, 12*, 23-38.

Laditka, S.B., & Laditka, J.N. (2001). Effects of improved morbidity rates on active life expectancy and eligibility for long-term care services. *Journal of Applied Gerontology, 10*, 39-56.

Laditka, S.B., & Wolf, D.A. (1998). New methods for analyzing active life expectancy. *Journal of Aging and Health, 10*, 214-241.

Land, K.C., Guralnik, J.M., & Blazer, D.G. (1994). Estimating increment-decrement life tables with multiple covariates from panel data: The case of active life expectancy. *Demography, 31*, 297-319.

Leveille, S.G., Penninx, B.W.J.H., Melzer, D., Izmirlian, G., & Guralnik, J.M. (2000). Sex differences in the prevalence of mobility disability in old age: The dynamics of incidence, recovery, and mortality. *Journal of Gerontology: Social Sciences, 55B*, S41-S50.

Manton, K.G. (1982). Changing concepts of morbidity and mortality in the elderly population. *Milbank Memorial Fund Quarterly, 60,* 183-191.

Manton, K.G., Corder, L., & Stallard, E. (1997). Chronic disability trends in the U.S. elderly populations 1982 to 1994, *Proceedings of the National Academy of Sciences, 94,* 2593-2598.

Manton, K.G., Corder, L., & Stallard, E. (1993). Estimates of change in chronic disability and institutional incidence and prevalence rates in the U.S. elderly population from the 1982, 1984, and 1989 National Long-Term Care Survey. *Journal of Gerontology: Social Sciences, 48,* S153-S166.

Manton, K.G., & Gu X. (2001). Changes in the prevalence of chronic disability in the United States black and nonblack population above age 65 from 1982 to 1999. *Proceedings of the National Academy of Sciences, 11,* 6354-6359.

Manton, K.G., & Stallard, E. (1997). Health and disability differences among racial and ethnic groups. In L.G. Martin & B.J. Soldo (Eds.), *Racial and ethnic differences in the health of older Americans* (pp. 43-105). Washington, DC: National Academy Press.

Manton, K.G., Woodbury, M.A., Stallard, E., & Corder, L.S. (1992). The use of grade of membership techniques to estimate regression relationships. *Sociological Methodology, 10,* 321-379.

Mathers, C.D., Murray, J.L., Lopez, A.D., Sadana, R., & Salomon, J.A. (2002). Global patterns of healthy life expectancy for older women. *Journal of Women & Aging, 14,* 168.

Matthews, K.A., Kelsey, S.F., Meilahn, E.N., Kuller, L.H., & Wing, R.R. (1989). Educational attainment and behavioral and biologic risk factors for coronary heart disease in middle age women. *American Journal of Epidemiology, 129,* 1132-1144.

Nusselder, W.J., van der Velden, K., van Sonsbeek, J.L.A., Lenior, M.E., & van den Bos, G.A.M. (1996). The elimination of selected chronic diseases in a population: The compression and expansion of morbidity. *American Journal of Public Health, 86,* 187-194.

Panapasa, S.V. (2002). Disability among older women and men in Fiji: Concerns for the future. *Journal of Women & Aging, 14,* 171.

Preston, S.H. (1992). Cohort succession and the future of the oldest old. In R. Suzman, D.P. Willis, & K.G. Manton (Eds.), *The oldest old* (pp. 50-57). New York: Oxford University Press.

Preston, S.H., Elo, I., Rosenwaike, I., & Hill, M. (1996). African American mortality at older ages: Results from a matching study. *Demography, 33,* 193-209.

Reed, D.M., Foley, D.J., White, L.R., Heimovitz, H., Burchfiel, C.M., & Masaki, K. (1998). Predictors of healthy aging in men with high life expectancies. *American Journal of Public Health, 88,* 1463-1468.

Robine, J.M., Jagger, C., & Cambois, E. (2002). European perspectives on healthy aging in women. *Journal of Women & Aging, 14,* 168.

Robine, J.M., Mormiche, P., & Sermet, C. (1998). Examination of the causes and mechanisms for the increase in disability-free life expectancy. *Journal of Aging and Health, 10,* 171-191.

Robine, J.M., & Ritchie, K. (1991). Healthy life expectancy: Evaluation of a global indicator of change in population health. *British Medical Journal, 302,* 457-460.

Robine, J.M., Romieu, I., & Cambois, E. (1997). Health expectancies and current research. *Reviews in Clinical Gerontology, 7*, 73-81.

Sauvaget, C., Tsuji, I., Aonuma, T., & Hisamichi, S. (1999). Health-life expectancy according to various functional levels. *Journal of the American Geriatrics Society, 47*, 1326-1331.

Schoeni, R.F., Freedman, V.A., & Wallace, R.B. (2001). Persistent, consistent, widespread, and robust? Another look at recent trends in old-age disability. *Journal of Gerontology: Social Sciences, 56B*, 206-S281.

Spiers, N., Jagger, C., & Clarke, M. (1996). Physical function and perceived health: Cohort differences and interrelationships in older people. *Journal of Gerontology: Social Sciences, 51B*, S226-S233.

Tsuji, I., Sauvaget, C., & Hisamichi, S. (2002). Health expectancies in Japan: Gender differences and policy implications for women. *Journal of Women & Aging, 14*, 168.

United States Census Bureau. (2000). International Database. Available at: http://www.census.gov/ipc/www/idbnew.html. Accessed July 23, 2001.

Vaupel, J.W., Carey, J.R., Christensen, K., Johnson, T.E., Yashin, A.I., Holm, N.V., Iachine, I.A., Kannisto, V., Khazaeli, A.A., Liedo, P., Longo, V.D., Zeng, Y., Manton, K.G., & Curtsinger, J.W. (1998). Biodemographic trajectories of longevity. *Science, 280*, 855-860.

Verbrugge, L.M. (1984). Longer life but worsening health? Trends in health and mortality of middle-aged and older persons. *Milbank Quarterly, 63*, 475-519.

Vita, A.J., Terry, R.B., Hubert, H.B., & Fries, J.F. (1998). Aging, health risks, and cumulative disability. *New England Journal of Medicine, 338*, 1035-1041.

Wachter, K.W., & Finch, C.E. (Eds.) (1997). *Between Zeus and the salmon: The biodemography of longevity.* Washington, DC: National Academy Press.

Waidmann, T.A., & Liu, K. (2000). Disability trends among elderly persons and implications for the future. *Journal of Gerontology: Social Sciences, 55B*, S298-S307.

Wister, A.V. (1996). Effects of socioeconomic status on exercise and smoking: Age-related differences. *Journal of Aging and Health, 8*, 467-488.

Wolf, D.A., Laditka, S.B., & Laditka, J.N. (2002). Patterns of active life among older women: Differences within and between groups. *Journal of Women & Aging, 14*, 171.

About the Contributors

Alain Bélanger, PhD, is Coordinator of the Research and Analysis Section at Statistics Canada. He also is the Editor of Statistics Canada's annual *Report on the Demographic Situation in Canada* and an Associate Researcher with the University of Quebec. Prior to his appointment with Statistics Canada, he worked as a researcher at the University of Quebec's *Institut National de la Recherche Scientifique* (INRS-Urbanization), at the International Institute for Applied System Analysis (IIASA) and at the University of Colorado. Dr. Bélanger's research interests include multi-state demography, healthy life expectancy, population aging and health, population migration, and population projections. He has authored and co-authored several papers in these fields, notably the first paper using multi-state modeling to estimate healthy life expectancy.

Jean-Marie Berthelot, BSc, has been the Manager of the Health Analysis and Modeling Group at Statistics Canada since 1991. He developed expertise in cancer economics through performing cost-of-illness and cost-effectiveness studies for lung, breast, and colorectal cancers. He is recognized as an expert in generic health status measures and their use in monitoring population health. He has co-authored many papers on the determinants of health. He is an investigator on several peer-reviewed grants and the principal investigator for the study of *Cohort mortality by socioeconomic characteristics: A mortality follow-up of 15% of the Canadian population,* funded by the Canadian Population Health Initiative. In 2001, he was awarded McMaster University's prestigious Labelle Lectureship in health services research.

Emmanuelle Cambois, PhD, is a researcher working in the Health and Demography team at the Department of Biostatistics, University of Montpellier 1, France. In the framework of the study of the health status of the population, she works on the measure of social differentials in mortality and health. She has computed disability-free life expectancy according to the occupational class for the French male population to assess the magnitude and trends in social differentials. Dr. Cambois is currently working on both the measure of inequalities in the disablement process and the measure of the mortality risks associated with life course pathways between occupational status.

Eileen M. Crimmins, PhD, is Edna M. Jones Professor of Gerontology and Sociology at the University of Southern California and Director of the University of Southern California/University of California at Los Angeles Center on Biodemography and Population Health, which is supported by the National Institute on Aging. She is currently working on two projects funded by the National Institute on Aging: The role of biological factors in educational and income differentials in health; and socioeconomic status differentials in active life expectancy in the older population. Dr. Crimmins is also working on the development of health indicators for assessing trends and differentials.

Dorly J. H. Deeg, PhD, MSc, is by education a methodologist, and has worked mainly in the areas of public health and gerontology. Since 1991, she has been appointed as Associate Professor of Social Epidemiology in the Vrije University Amsterdam, Department of Psychiatry, and in the Institute of Research in Extramural Medicine. She is also the Scientific Director of the Longitudinal Aging Study Amsterdam. Dr. Deeg is a Fellow of the Gerontological Society of America. Her publications include studies of chronic conditions, functional limitations, cognitive decline, depression and anxiety disorders, personal competence, limitations, social support, and methodological issues.

Aaron Hagedorn, BS, is a PhD student in Gerontology at the University of Southern California, where he also completed a dual Master of Science program in Gerontology and Health Administration. He has conducted research on gender differences in carpal tunnel syndrome and cross-national differences in chronic health conditions in the United States and Japan. He is a Research Assistant in the University of Southern California/University of California at Los Angeles Center on Biodemography and Population Health.

Shigeru Hisamichi, MD, PhD, received an MD in 1963 and a PhD in 1968 from Tohoku University School of Medicine, Sendai, Japan. Since 1981, he has been a Professor at the Department of Public Health, Tohoku University School of Medicine. He was the Dean of Tohoku University School of Medicine from 1995 to 2001. He was the Chairman of the Public Health Council for the Ministry of Health and Welfare in Japan from 1998 to 2000. Dr. Hisamichi has published numerous monographs and articles on cancer screening, epidemiological evaluation of health policy programs, and gerontology.

Carol Jagger, PhD, is an epidemiologist with a background in medical statistics and is Professor of Epidemiology in the Department of Epidemiology and Public Health at the University of Leicester, England. Her main research area is in gerontology, particularly the mental and physical health of older people; much of this work was undertaken with an ongoing longitudinal study, the Melton Mowbray Ageing Project. Dr. Jagger has been an active member of the International Network on Health Expectancy (REVES) since 1992, has been on the steering committee of both of the European REVES projects and also participated in the EURODEM project "Monitoring Neurodegenerative Disease of Public Health Importance in Europe."

Jung Ki Kim, PhD, is a Postdoctoral Fellow at the Andrus Gerontology Center of the University of Southern California. She received a PhD in Gerontology/Public Policy at the University of Southern California. Her dissertation was on the effect of marital status on health outcomes among older people, particularly how different marital status, changes of marital status, duration of widowhood, and living arrangements affect health outcomes. Dr. Kim's current and future research interests include work on health and other risk adjustment among Medicare and Medicaid populations.

James N. Laditka, DA, MPA, is a PhD candidate in Public Administration and a Research Associate of the Center for Policy Research at Syracuse University. Dr. Laditka's research interests are health services research and gerontology, including utilization of formal and informal health care, the demography of aging, and health policy. Dr. Laditka's published research includes studies of healthy life expectancy, health care resource utilization, home and community based services, family caregiving, both long-term care and acute care services, and preventable hospitalization.

Sarah B. Laditka, PhD, is Associate Professor of Health Services Management and Director of the Center for Health and Aging at the State University of New York Institute of Technology. Her previous positions include Manager of Health Programs at the General Electric Company. Dr. Laditka's publications include studies on active life expectancy, quality of life for older individuals, utilization of health services for special populations, access to primary health care services, family caregiving, and utilization and satisfaction with long-term care services.

Maarten Lindeboom, PhD, is Professor of Economics in the Department of Economics of the Vrije University, Amsterdam, and Director of Graduate Studies of the Tinbergen Institute in The Netherlands. His is also a Research Fellow of the Tinbergen Institute and at the Institut für die Zukunft der Arbeit in Bonn, Germany. His research interests include labor economics, the incentive effects of social security, labor force participation behavior of older persons, and the dynamic interrelation between work, income and health, sickness absenteeism, and survey non-response and attrition in longitudinal surveys.

Alan D. Lopez, PhD, is the Coordinator for the Epidemiology and Burden of Disease program at the World Health Organization (WHO) in Geneva, Switzerland. He was coauthor, with Christopher Murray, MD, of the groundbreaking Global Burden of Disease Study and has published extensively on global mortality, epidemiology, and the assessment of health risk factors.

Laurent Martel, MSc, is a demographer and a Senior Analyst at the Demography Division of Statistics Canada. He joined Statistics Canada in 1997 after working as a research analyst at the *Institut National d'Études Démographiques (INED)* in Paris and at the United Nations Economic Commission for Europe (UNECE) in Geneva, Switzerland. He is also a member of the board of directors of the *Association Internationale des Démographes de Langue Française*. His main research interests are population aging and health indicators. He has published many articles on living arrangements, social support, and transitions between functional health states among the elderly and, more recently, on disability-free life expectancy.

Colin D. Mathers, PhD, works for the Global Program on Evidence for Health Policy at the World Health Organization (WHO) in Geneva, Switzerland. His main responsibilities are the analysis of healthy life expectancy and the revision of the Global Burden of Disease for non-communicable diseases. Dr. Mathers has authored and co-authored numerous publications on the measurement of population health trends and differentials, with a particular emphasis on health expectancies and other summary measures of health that combine morbidity and mortality. Prior to joining WHO, Dr. Mathers was Principal Research Fellow at the Australian Institute of Health and Welfare, where he carried out the first study of the burden of disease and injury in Australia.

Fiona Matthews, MSc, has been the Project Statistician for the Cognitive Function and Aging Study since 1997, and is affiliated with the Medical Research Council Biostatistics Unit in Cambridge, England. She has a varied role within the study investigating many areas, including the healthy active life expectancy field, but is also involved in analysis of neuropathology and incidence estimation techniques. Prior to coming to Cambridge, she worked as a statistician in Cancer Research in Surrey.

Christopher J. L. Murray, MD, is Executive Director for Evidence and Information for Policy at the World Health Organization (WHO). Trained in medicine and economics, he has written and co-authored over 100 publications on a wide array of health issues. Dr. Murray's key priority at WHO is developing a framework to assess, monitor, and evaluate the performance of health systems. This has led to the development of tools to measure the performance of health systems, and on subsequent work with policy makers to develop ways of improving performance based on the results. Prior to joining WHO, Dr. Murray was Professor of International Health Economics and Director of the Burden of Disease Unit at Harvard University.

Sela V. Panapasa, PhD, is a National Institute on Aging Postdoctoral Research Fellow with the Population Studies Center, Institute for Social Research at the University of Michigan in Ann Arbor. She received a PhD in Sociology from Brown University. Dr. Panapasa is a social demographer who studies family support and intergenerational exchanges among the elderly in Fiji. Her interests also include examining the welfare of Pacific Island families relative to the ongoing changes throughout the region. Dr. Panapasa's more recent work looks at health issues of aging and elderly well-being in Fiji.

France Portrait, PhD, studied quantitative economics and econometrics at the University of Aix-Marseille (France). She began working on her dissertation at the Department of Econometrics of the Vrije University, Amsterdam, in 1995. The subject of her dissertation is the use of long-term care services by the Dutch elderly. Currently, Dr. Portrait is a Postdoctoral Fellow at Vrije University, in the Department of Econometrics.

Jean-Marie Robine, DED, is a Senior Research Fellow at the French National Institute of Health and Medical Research and head of the *Health and Demography* team at the Department of Biostatistics, University of Montpellier 1, France. His research focuses on measuring the impact that the continuation of increases in life expectancy may have on the health status of the population. In particular, he works on the measure of disability and on the evolution of the health status of populations. He also studies human longevity, with the aim of understanding the relations between health and longevity. Since its creation in 1989, Dr. Robine has been the coordinator of the International Network on Health Expectancy (REVES), which brings together more than 150 researchers from more than 100 research establishments in over 30 countries worldwide.

Ritu Sadana, PhD, is a scientist within the World Health Organization (WHO) Global Program on Evidence for Health Policy. She has an extensive background in the measurement and description of health status, with a particular interest in the use of health survey data for comparison of the health of populations, and has responsibility for the analysis of data from the WHO survey program.

Joshua A. Salomon, PhD, works within the World Health Organization (WHO) Global Program on Evidence for Health Policy on health state valuation methods and analyses. He is also involved in the global burden of disease project with a particular focus on the estimation of disability weights and of the projection of the global burden of disease in the future.

Catherine Sauvaget, MD, PhD, received an MD in 1992 from Rennes University School of Medicine, in France, and a PhD in 1998 from Tohoku University School of Medicine, Sendai, Japan. She was an Assistant Professor at the Department of Public Health, Tohoku University School of Medicine from 1998 to 2000. She is now a Research Scientist at the Department of Epidemiology, the Radiation Effects Research Foundation, Hiroshima, Japan. Dr. Sauvaget has published many articles on dementia-free and disability-free life expectancies. Her current research areas include risk factors of functional disability, and the relationship between cognition and functional performances.

Ichiro Tsuji, MD, PhD, received an MD in 1983 and a PhD in 1991 from Tohoku University School of Medicine, Sendai, Japan. He was a Research Fellow at The Johns Hopkins University School of Hygiene from 1991 to 1993. Dr. Tsuji is an Associate Professor at the Department of Public Health, Tohoku University School of Medicine. He has published many articles in journals on geriatrics and gerontology. He is a co-author of the monograph *Intergenerational Programs: Support for Children, Youth, and Elders in Japan.* His current research areas include epidemiology of aging, impact of lifestyle upon medical costs, and randomized trials for disability prevention among elderly individuals.

Russell Wilkins, MUrb, is a Senior Analyst with the Health Analysis and Modeling Group at Statistics Canada, and Adjunct Professor of Epidemiology and Community Medicine at the University of Ottawa. His main research interests are socioeconomic inequalities in mortality and birth outcomes, and summary measures of population health expectancy using vital statistics, survey, and administrative data. Russell began his career in population health at the Institute for Research on Public Policy in Montreal (1978-83), then moved to the Montreal General Hospital Department of Community Health (1983-87), before joining Statistics Canada in 1988. He is on the editorial boards of *Les Cahiers Québécois de Démographie* and the *International Journal for Equity in Health,* and was a founding member of the International Network on Health Expectancy (REVES).

Douglas A. Wolf, PhD, is a demographer, policy analyst, program evaluator, and gerontological researcher who studies the economic, demographic, and social aspects of aging and long-term care. Dr. Wolf's professional experience includes an appointment as an economist in the Department of Health and Human Services' Office of Income Security Policy and several years at the Urban Institute. He is currently Professor of Public Administration, Gerald B. Cramer Professor of Aging Studies, and Associate Director of the Maxwell School's Center for Policy Research at Syracuse University. Dr. Wolf's research areas include several topics in the well-being and life-course patterns of the older population, such as household composition and parent-child coresidence; the dynamics of nursing home use; use of community-based, long-term care resources; and the spatial distribution of kin and migration choices.

Index